THE SUPER CARB DIET

ALSO BY BOB HARPER

Are You Ready!

The Skinny Rules

Jumpstart to Skinny

Skinny Meals

Skinny Habits

THE SUPER CARB DIET

BOB HARPER

with Danny Pellegrino

ST. MARTIN'S PRESS ⋙ NEW YORK

THE SUPER CARB DIET. Copyright © 2017 by Bob Harper. All rights reserved. Printed in the United States of America. For information, address St. Martin's Press, 175 Fifth Avenue, New York, N.Y. 10010.

www.stmartins.com

Book design by Richard Oriolo

The Library of Congress Cataloging-in-Publication Data
is available upon request.

ISBN 978-1-250-14660-1 (hardcover)
ISBN 978-1-250-14661-8 (ebook)

Our books may be purchased in bulk for promotional, educational, or business use. Please contact your local bookseller or the Macmillan Corporate and Premium Sales Department at 1-800-221-7945, extension 5442, or by email at MacmillanSpecialMarkets@macmillan.com.

First Edition: December 2017

10 9 8 7 6 5 4 3 2 1

I am dedicating this book to Cristi Conaway, Kate Angelo, Nicole Trinler, Anthony Gutierrez, Kelsey Johnson, and Debbie Johnson. They were the angels that were there for me during the hardest time of my life. When I awoke from the heart attack that left me unconscious for two days, they were right by my bedside. I will be forever grateful to them for showing me unconditional love when I needed it most. My heart may have been broken, but they made sure it was full.

CONTENTS

PREFACE
The Super Carb Catalyst

February 12, 2017, is a day I don't remember, at all, and a day I won't ever forget. I died that day, a Sunday, in a gym in my Chelsea, New York, neighborhood. Sounds dramatic, but it's very much a true story.

The last thing I remember is having an early dinner with my friend Sean and his boyfriend that Saturday night. We had an early meal because we were planning to meet the next morning at Brick New York, a CrossFit gym where we work out regularly. I left them after dinner, walked home, took my dog, Karl, for a short walk, and then went to bed. What follows is the story of what happened the next day, as told to me by Sean and the other people who were there.

Sunday morning, I walked to the gym with my dog and met up with Sean for our workout. Sean told me that I was complaining about being dizzy as soon as I arrived. A little backstory: About six weeks prior to this day I was in Los Angeles and I fainted in the middle of a workout. I had never experienced anything like that in all my years of working out. I felt incredibly dizzy, and the next thing I knew I was being awakened by a couple of friends in the group class. I figured I had worked out too hard that day, or maybe it was because I didn't have anything to eat prior to the class. Whatever the case, I didn't take it too seriously. In the weeks leading up to my heart attack, I was experiencing similar dizzy spells, although I didn't faint. At the gym, I would reprogram workouts, adjusting the movements that would make me feel off. I would change to lighter weights to adapt as needed. Basically, I was just doing these things to try to avoid the dizzy spells instead of figuring out the root cause of my problem. I was breaking a cardinal rule I have been preaching for my whole career. I was NOT listening to my body. The dizzy spells were becoming more consistent and a growing concern of mine, so I went to a doctor, who suggested I get some further tests done. I put these tests off. Some friends suggested I try taking Dramamine. Unfortunately, that didn't help.

Okay, so now let's get back to that Sunday morning. Sean told me I was already complaining about being dizzy. We started the workout. It was brutal, but no more so than usual. Sean finished before me and took a seat on the floor afterward to recover from the grueling exercise. He said that he looked over at me and I stopped in the middle of the workout, which is odd because it is very unlike me to stop entirely. Then he saw me get down on the floor and lie on my side. He asked me if I was feeling dizzy, and I nodded my head to say "yes." Then I rolled on my back. Sean was smart enough to know that something wasn't right. He came over to me and saw that I was completely unresponsive. He rushed to turn the music off, immediately told our coach, Sherry, that I had passed out, and then got someone to call 911. Sherry ran upstairs where the AED (Automated External Defibrillator) was located. An event was going on upstairs, so she asked if there was a doctor in the house—literally—and guess what? There was. A man named Hazem Shoirah, who wasn't even a member of the gym. Dr. Shoirah ran downstairs and saw me on the floor where someone was performing CPR on me. He stepped in and took over CPR as Sherry got the AED attached to me. The AED initially did not perform because I was in what is called asystole, which basically means I flatlined. Dr. Shoirah told me two months later that this was the point at which he got "concerned." My heart had stopped and my lips turned blue, but he didn't stop perform-ing CPR. On the second attempt the AED delivered a shock, but I was still in cardiac arrest. The paramedics showed up at this point, very quickly from what I was told, and they took over. They pulled out their heavy-duty defibrillators and gave me a shock that was so intense, Sherry, the fitness coach, said that my whole body levitated off the floor. Off the floor! This still gives me chills. This was all happening to ME! How in the world was this fucking hap-pening to ME?!

The paramedics got my heart going, but I was still uncon-scious. They got me in the ambulance as fast as they could and rushed me to the emergency room at Mount Sinai Beth Israel. My assistant, Nicole, arrived about ten minutes after I did. She was sent into the room to talk to the team that was working on me. The doctors moved me to the cath lab where they put the first of two stents into my heart (the second one followed in the days after I woke up from the coma). This procedure took about an hour and a half. After they were finished, they moved me to the cardiac intensive care unit. There they started the process of therapeutic hypothermia, a process where they literally put me on ice and in an induced coma to protect me from any brain damage that I might have experienced from the time (which is unclear to me, but estimated around seven to twelve minutes) that my brain was without oxygen. The entire time I was in the hospital, Nicole became the voice I didn't have. She contacted my sister and niece, and my closest friends from Los Angeles to tell them what had happened. Everyone was on the next plane to New York City.

For two whole days I was in a coma induced by my doctors. When I woke up, I was surrounded by my closest friends and family, but let me tell you, I was SUPER confused. Imagine losing two whole days of your life! They told me what had happened and I proceeded to get very emotional, but the crazy part is that I was experiencing short-term memory loss. About every ten minutes I would look around and get confused all over again. I would ask the same things over and over—what happened, why am I here, and why are you all here? I felt like Dory from *Finding Nemo*.

For eight days and seven nights, the hospital was my home. Eight *very* long days. I have never wanted to leave a place so badly in my entire life. I wanted to go home to my bed in my cozy New York City apartment. The nurses took such great care of me at the hospital. I'm so thankful for them and everyone who helped me through my stay at Mount Sinai Beth Israel. They even turned a blind eye when my friends brought my dog, Karl, to the hospital to be with me. I tear up right now just thinking about how he visited me when I needed him most. My friends, Cristi, Kate, Anthony,

Nicole, Debbie, and Kelsey also came through, never leaving me alone while I was there. I am forever grateful for that. Despite the love, I was ready to get back to my real home.

When I finally did get to leave the hospital, all I could do was rest. The first time I left the house, I thought I would be able to go for a walk around the block to get some fresh air. I made it halfway before I had to turn back and get home. Me, the fitness guy who works out every day, could not walk around the block without getting winded or dizzy. It was a humbling experience, to say the least. Humbling and tough. Speaking of tough, did I mention that I developed pneumonia during my hospital stay? I was in constant pain. The pneumonia had me coughing and my chest was still so tender from the CPR that was performed on me. The chest pain was tough, but I thank God that I was around to experience that pain.

The next couple of months after my heart attack, when I was home recovering, were very emotional. I battled depression, which won the fight on most days. "My heart gave up on me," repeated in my head. Rationally, I knew this was crazy, but I couldn't stop it. My heart had been pumping away in my chest without any problems for years. It kept me running around as a kid all the way through my adulthood. It beat perfectly as I worked on a farm all those long, hot summers of my youth. I spent endless nights dancing at concerts and dance clubs without any problems. My heart swelled as I fell in love, and survived brutal breakups throughout my fifty-one years. It even helped me through countless agonizing workouts. But on February 12, 2017, it just stopped.

I've cried a lot over my broken heart since that February day. Now that it's recovered I am trying to trust it again. The cardiac rehab program I did helped me through all these feelings. The professionals had me doing workouts that I would have scoffed at before, but found myself embracing. The very first time I went to rehab, I was scared. I kept feeling like I would finish the workout they had planned for me, then go home and drop dead from another heart attack. Not only that, but I didn't have the safety net of a hospital stay after that first session. I would go home to my apartment and be all alone. When I was in the hospital, I couldn't wait to get out, but when I was back home, I longed for professional supervision. It was terrifying. My physical therapists at rehab had to talk me off the ledge that I was standing on inside my head. They reminded me I had to start trusting my heart again, that day and every day thereafter. My heart and I are still building that trust. That is why I am doing everything I can possibly do to give my heart what it needs. That means proper nutrition daily. And rest. And smart and effective exercise and stress management. Yoga is really helping me with that. I said on the *Today* show when I shared my story that I was not going to stress over the little things or the big things anymore. I said I would focus on the things that really matter in life. Friends. Family. My dog. Love. Happiness. My goal now is practicing what I preach, and this time I am.

The type of heart attack I had is called a widowmaker. It was caused primarily by a genetic condition I have, high lipoprotein(a), or Lp(a), a particle in the blood that carries cholesterol, fat, and proteins and is inherited from your parents. I knew heart problems ran in my family, and I encourage you all to find out if they run in yours, too. If you don't know your family's health history, do a little digging. If you have older relatives who are alive, ask them. Call up your mom or dad and ask if they, or either set of grandparents, ever had heart problems. It's a quick conversation that can make a huge difference. Once you know, always be sure to tell your primary physician. If your doctor knows, that person can monitor your health as it relates to your heart health.

Doctors have since told me the survival rate of a widowmaker is 6 to 10 percent. That statistic will haunt me for the rest of my life. I'll never be able to forget how lucky I was to survive what could've been the end of the road for me. Fortunately, it wasn't. I survived, and I survived, I believe, because I still have more to do. I have more to teach and more change to make in the world. Everyone out there reading this right now must know of someone who has had a heart attack. Sometimes, yes, it is related to your eating habits or your exercise routine. But for others, like me, it had nothing to do with those factors.

I've always had a healthy diet and a regimented exercise routine. And what I've been told by the many wonderful doctors that have cared for me since my heart attack is that I wouldn't have survived and recovered so well if it weren't for how healthy I live my life. Hopefully, you will never enter cardiac arrest. If you do, I want you all to be strong enough to fight that battle and more. Whether it's heart problems, diabetes, obesity, the flu, or any other ailments that may be presented to you, I want you to have the tools you need to survive and heal. I've had teams of doctors giving me diet advice and exercise plans. One of my doctors, Dean Ornish, M.D., is brilliant, and he formulated a diet plan that I followed immediately after the attack. It started out vegetarian, really watching my fat intake. Slowly, I incorporated more nonfat plain Greek yogurt and egg whites into my nutritional regimen. Then other foods followed.

I've used the information Dean Ornish and other doctors

taught me, along with everything I've learned in all my years in the health-and-fitness industry, to craft the very best, well-rounded diet plan for all of you. This plan will help you lose weight and keep you healthy. It's not just for people with heart problems. The Super Carb Diet is for everyone. My focus has become not just weight loss, but doing it without sacrificing the rest of your health. My life-threatening experience has only deepened my understanding of both the body and the mind. I've learned to embrace foods and philosophies I didn't always subscribe to in my previous years. Strict is good, but balance is key. The diet plan I created is all about being strict and finding that balance. I bet you're wondering what that means. For you, it means ninety days. Ninety days of hard work. Ninety days of:

1. **FOOD.** Three square and BALANCED meals per day, plus one "floater" meal. We're going to balance the plate to fit YOU. That means creating a meal plan based on your weight and your goals. Before this book is finished, you'll have a meal plan that is specific to YOU. You will learn what those meals entail and how to get your numbers shortly, but know that you'll be eating protein, fat, AND carbs. That's right, carbs. After all, it's called the Super Carb Diet for a reason.

2. **SLEEP.** We're going to get the proper rest on this diet because your body needs it.

3. **FITNESS.** You'll be active on this plan, so go buy a durable water bottle and a pair of workout shoes.

4. **ACCOUNTABILITY.** I'm talking about weighing your food and yourself. This diet is all about numbers. In the kitchen, on the scale, and in your food journals.

Gone are the days of no carbs. Your body needs what it needs, so this plan is about giving you what it needs. I'm going to get you as healthy as I possibly can so you can survive whatever comes your way. Not only that, but it's going to make you look and feel better than you ever have. They say everything happens for a reason. My heart attack happened, and I spent so much time searching for the reason. The Super Carb Diet is part of that reason. *This* is why I'm part of that 6-to-10 percent. I now have a passion to help people more than ever in my life, and that is exactly what I am doing. Right here. Right now.

INTRODUCTION
Body by Bob

CARB. For many of us, "carb" is the most terrifying of all the four-letter words. We've given it so much power throughout the years that it's impossible to think about carbohydrates with any sort of objectivity. I'm here to change that. Not only that, but I'm here to put them back on your plate and get the power back.

Carbohydrates do not make you fat. They are defined as "any one of various substances found in certain foods (such as bread, rice, and potatoes) that provide your body with heat and energy and are made of carbon, hydrogen, and oxygen."[1] So why does society seem to define them as "the enemy"? Carbs don't make you fat! Let me repeat, carbs provide *heat* and *energy*. It's right there in the definition. You know where else you're going to find carbs? On a balanced plate of food. At fifty-one years old, after a heart attack no less, I needed balance. And so do you.

Throughout all my years on *The Biggest Loser*, I've seen and heard it all when it comes to weight loss. Many contestants come on the show for one reason, and one reason only: to lose weight. But it isn't just *TBL* contestants. I still train clients at every single fitness level and find them searching for the same answers. Aside from my clients, there are people who have never worked out a day in their lives as well as athletes who have trained for years asking me what they can do to drop weight. It doesn't matter if you're a stay-at-home dad who can't fit into the minivan, a single thirty-one-year-old looking to drop a few pounds before taking your dating profile picture, or a twentysomething girl looking to compete at the CrossFit Games. We all want to better our bodies and ourselves. But what is the best way to do it?

Fad diets have come and gone and, at fifty-one years old, I've done my fair share. After my heart attack, I was searching for a way to balance my diet without gaining weight. I needed a diet high in nutrients that would help me maintain my weight and give me the energy I needed to recover. Not only that, but it's my job to stay on top of what's going on in the world of health and fitness, and I'm damn good at my job. *The Biggest Loser* started in 2004, and thirteen years later I am still standing. I've even written books about breaking your habits and following rules. I stand by everything I've said in those books, while also understanding that fitness and nutrition are constantly evolving. The dieting world went back in time to find variations of the caveman diet, but I found those high-protein plans had too much fat and weren't so great for my heart. They didn't work for me. They left my body off balance.

As trends have changed, I've experimented. Throughout my experimentation, there was one constant: no carbs after a specific time. Trendy diets tell you that you can't have carbs. But I want bread. So does Oprah. So do you. I want to eat a sandwich at lunch without feeling like I'm committing a crime. Did you know a sandwich isn't a sandwich unless there's bread? So, I started looking for a plan that allowed me the heat and energy I need to work out, to sleep well, and to have the mental capacity to go about my busy day. When I didn't find a plan, I began to formulate one with my doctors around the exact thing everyone fears—carbohydrates.

To formulate the plan, I had to experiment a bit more. I reset my thinking and went back to basics. I had the best doctors in the world giving me different advice. I took it all in. I also got friends involved. Friends that knew about balance. Friends like Nick Shaw, CEO of Renaissance Periodization, and Karianne Anthes, (CF-L4), owner of CrossFit Morristown, CF HQ Seminar Staff, who showed me that a balanced meal meant more than just protein and fat. They helped me understand that we can craft a diet for people trying to lose weight, for people who want to maintain weight, and even for those super-athletes who want to put on weight. It sounds like an impossibility, but it's not. Not when it becomes a game of numbers. These friends showed me a whole new world of turning my plate into a math equation. Every meal became about counting and balancing. Remember that food pyramid we all learned about in grade school? I looked at that triangle and thought about what foods my body needed, what foods my body didn't need, and how they fit into each meal. I needed to figure out what foods, and how much, would provide me with the mental and physical strength I was looking for to get me through my hectic day AND get back to optimum health. One thing that stuck with me when I looked at that food pyramid was the large base filled with bread, rice, pasta, and cereal. I wanted some of *that* again, but I needed to reorganize it.

The desire for spaghetti, wild rice, and a baguette led me to slowly reintroduce carbs into my diet. When I did, I felt guilty and scared. It had been so long since I embraced them! It's not just me. We're all brainwashed into thinking that we will get fat if we have carbs. Seriously, I was terrified to eat even a morsel of anything carb-based because it had been uncharted territory. Suddenly a rice bowl with veggies and chicken felt like I was bingeing on Halloween candy. I've been doing this my whole life. I know better, and I STILL second-guessed myself every time a grain went in my mouth. Why? Because everyone tells us carbohydrates are bad. Not just bad, but cheat-meal territory. It was as if I should only be eating a carb on a holiday. But, remember, carbs don't make you fat. I'm here to tell you that's unequivocally false, so Merry Carby Christmas! Of course, there are plenty of garbage carbs out there, or as I like to call them, "carbage," but there are also some great ones. I'll teach you how to spot the difference.

The Super Carb Diet isn't JUST about eating carbs, so don't start buttering your toast just yet. We're also going to talk about the type and amount of protein and fat you need on your plate, with an emphasis on the veggies. I'm going to make sure you get the right amount of everything to create a balanced meal at *every* meal. Your plate is going to start to look like a beautiful and delicious math equation. That means giving up a lot of foods you may love, and discovering foods that may be new to you. I love a chocolate chip cookie just as much as the next guy, but it doesn't have a place in my weight-loss plan. So forget it. You'll be able to have a cookie again, but right now I want you to be strict. I'm going to be your weight loss GPS, so just listen to where I'm telling you to go, and I promise you'll get results. You picked up or downloaded this book to lose weight, so I'm not going to sugarcoat it. Nothing will be coated with sugar in the near future, so get used to it.

So now, here's where I scare you. Weight loss is not easy. If it were, we wouldn't have the obesity problems we do in America. According to the National Institutes of Health, the second leading cause of preventable death in the United States is obesity.[2] The dollar menu is affordable and convenient, I get it. Guess what? I don't care. If you pay now for the foods that are going to get you healthy, you won't have to pay in doctor bills later. And doctor bills are expensive! You either pay now, or you pay later. I want you to lose weight and I want to teach you realistic ways to do it. I'm letting you have carbs, so don't get mad at me because you can't have the sugar or cheat meals you want. Want to know what's even harder than weight loss? Maintaining the weight after you've lost it. This plan will help you do it, but YOU must make the commitment. YOU must put in the work. I'm here to guide you. I showed up and wrote this book, so it's time for you to show up and give it a try. One thing I want to let you know up front, is that it will NOT be easy. I know you all want a simple fix, and if there was one, I promise I would be writing about that instead because it would probably sell a helluva lot more books to people looking for an easy way out. But you know what? My way will be worth it. Like anything that is hard, I promise you will feel a sense of accomplishment when you start to change your workout routine and your diet plan, just like I did. Most importantly, you'll get results. If you're not seeing changes in your body with your current routine, then now is as good as a time as any to try something new. Just give me ninety days.

The Super Carb Diet worked for me. My body needed a reset. The old tricks weren't working, so I had to go back to square one. Crash diets where you consume nothing but water and lemon all day are no longer an option. I got a second chance at life when I survived that heart attack, so I don't have any chances left. If you want to lose or maintain your weight, you must do it in a balanced way or you will compromise your overall health. I found that this plan wasn't *just* working on my fifty-one-year-old body. Once it started working for me, I began to share it with the people I love most. Soon, it began to work for them. People in their twenties and people in their sixties found success. Friends that wanted to gain weight used the equation to do so in a healthy way. Have a wedding coming up and you want to lose weight for it? The plan works for that, too. The Super Carb Diet began to help friends manage weight and feel better about themselves. When I saw the physical and mental changes happening not just for me, but those around me, I knew I had to share the Super Carb Diet with the world. In all my years of teaching health and fitness, this is the most effective method I've found for people to lose weight and maintain their overall health. It's not just about weight loss. It's about strength. It's about fuel. We're using carbs to fuel your day. I'm giving you the gas you need to power through your next workout. You didn't think I was going to forget about the workout, did you? Your workouts are going to feel great because you'll be giving your body the proper nutrients to be successful in the gym. My workouts are going to help sculpt your body into the body you've always dreamed of. Diet and exercise go together like the peanut butter and jelly that are going between the two slices of bread you're going to be eating. But for you to be successful in the gym, I need you to be successful in the kitchen first.

So, pour yourself some coffee because I'm going to teach you about good carbs, bad carbs, and everything in between, doing my best to make it clear and easy to understand. When I set out to write this book, I thought about what to include. I decided that you need the same tools I do. This is the book I wish I had when I set out to reintroduce carbs into my life. I'll share a sample food journal, sample menus, and some recipes that worked for me so you'll have some meal ideas. These are the recipes I cooked again and again until I perfected them. The recipes are balanced and full of fuel for our bodies. If you follow me on Instagram (@bobharper), you know I'm constantly bragging (#ImAChef) about my food. I share because I'm proud, and it tastes GOOD. Now you'll get a chance to try my food and hopefully you'll share your results with me (#SuperCarbDiet).

People come up to me on the street all the time and ask me questions about health and fitness. There are a handful of questions I get CONSTANTLY. Questions like, "How do I lose the last five pounds?" or, "Should I weigh myself every day?" Number one on that list? "What's the healthiest alcohol?" Everyone wants to know. You may be wondering, "Can I have alcohol on this diet?" No. But I did dedicate a whole section to that question so you can have a handy guide with you when you absolutely cannot not have a cocktail. Again, I'm not saying you can drink on this diet, but I'll give you the tools for you to factor it in if you do. We'll get into that later. I wanted to include the info on the booze and other frequently asked questions so that long after you've completed this program and gotten the body you dreamed of, you can keep this book on your shelf and pull it out when you need it. When you're going out with friends to splurge, you can open the alcohol chapter and craft some healthy cocktails that are Bob-approved and carb-friendly, right alongside those food recipes.

Food isn't all I share on social media. You'll also notice I showcase my workouts quite often. Annoying, right? Well, it's not all about taking a shirtless selfie for "likes." I teach Body by Bob in New York and LA to a diverse clientele, some of the fittest athletes in the world alongside people at the gym for the very first time. Why do people keep coming back? Because of my programming. I share these workouts because they are crafted with YOU in mind. They are challenges that anyone can do and everyone can benefit from. In this book, I'll share some of those workout plans so you can do your own Body by Bob from home or at your nearest house of fitness. These workouts are movements that I've tested at my Body by Bob classes, on *The Biggest Loser*, and in my own daily life. They are what I've found to be *the* most successful after years of trial and error. I even included a few of my rehab workouts for those of you recovering alongside me. I've never included rehabilitation workouts in any of my books, but I realized that some of you, for a variety of reasons, may need them. So, they're here. There are workouts you can do at home with no equipment, at the gym with lots of equipment, and even some you can do in a hotel room when you travel. The food you make in the kitchen will be the gas you need to get through any of my workouts. Let this book be your workbook and the food be your fuel.

I want you to believe in yourself because I believe in you. You may be thinking you don't deserve the body you want, but I'm here to tell you that you do. We all do. I must believe that, otherwise why would I have devoted my entire life's work to making people fit and healthy? Money is great, but it will not put you to sleep at night (that said, a good mattress and some high-thread-count sheets will help you sleep, but I digress). I do what I do because I love it. Seeing people change the way they eat and the way they live helps me sleep at night. It keeps me warm when the mattress and sheets aren't working.

What I've seen after all these years is that many of you are afraid of success when it comes to your bodies. You feel you don't deserve it. You *do*. Every time you think you might quit or give up on this plan, I want you to circle back to me and remember that you do deserve it. That I believe in you. I'm giving you some of the love that I want you to put back on your plate.

The Super Carb Diet is a passion project of mine. A friend of mine likes to say that everyone needs a "slumpbuster," or something to jump-start a new path, whether it is in relationship patterns or eating habits. Carbs were my slumpbuster, and they led me to the Super Carb Diet. I want you to look at this book as everything you need to be successful and get out of your slump. Let me be your slumpbuster.

After years on *The Biggest Loser* and training people outside of the show, I've learned what other people want and need to be successful in their physical transformation. They want no-nonsense. I get it, believe me, I get it. I want no-nonsense, too. That's why I'm going to tell you exactly what to do in the kitchen and the gym. No more guessing. I'm taking the guessing out of it. You'll know exactly how much you're consuming every time you eat. It will take discipline on your end, some investing (food scale, anyone?), and trust. I need you to trust me. Trust that I have your best interest at heart. I want you to succeed. Not only for my own reputation, but because I want you to be happy. I want you to be satisfied. If you're happy, that means you'll come up to me on the street, or tweet me (@MyTrainerBob) and tell me how much you liked my plan and what you've learned about carbs. You'll walk around with a smile on your face and fill the world up with just a little bit more love. Remember when I told you that I want you to put some love on your plate? Well, I need it, too. Your success will help me fill my plate. So let's get started!

PART I

THE SUPER CARB DIET RULES

1.

CARBS DON'T
MAKE YOU FAT

Carbs don't make you fat. After all my years in the industry, I find this to be one of the biggest misconceptions when it comes to weight loss. So many people think carbs equal fat. That's wrong. Completely wrong. I hate to be so harsh, but every now and then we need a little tough love. While it's true that carbs can be dangerous if you're overeating or not eating the right ones, they *do* have a place in your daily life. In fact, The American Society for Nutrition published a study in February 2017 that found that switching to a diet with whole grains appeared to lower the number of calories absorbed by the body during digestion and speed up your metabolism.[1] Those whole grains are carbs, and it's proof they're not all bad. From now on, I want you to think of fuel. I want you to think about fuel every time you hear the word "carb." If you're going to start changing the way you eat, I need you to start changing the way you think. It starts with knowing that carbs will fuel your body and mind. Good carbs are going to give you the energy you need to get through your next workout and, more generally, through your day. By ingesting a healthy amount of good carbohydrates, you're giving your body the fuel it needs to be successful. How exactly is it fueled? Glucose.

Our brains and bodies run on glucose. It's the most important source of energy our body has. Coffee is great, but unless you hook an espresso IV to your vein, java beans won't be able to energize you long-term. Glucose is the energy we need, and we get glucose from carbohydrates. This is where things get a little complicated, so bear with me. Carbs, originally made up of sugar and starch, are broken down into glucose when the stomach digests them. That means every time you put a carb in your mouth, the process of turning it into glucose begins. Once broken down, the stomach and small intestine absorb that glucose, where it is either immediately used for energy or stored for later use. Since glucose is the main source of energy, our body needs carbohydrates to successfully power its engine.

Let's break this down even further: carbs are molecules made up of hydrogen, carbon, and oxygen atoms. Stay with me. Each carbohydrate is composed of one of three monosaccharides. Monosaccharides is a fancy way of saying sugar. Still there? I know this is a lot of scientific information, but it's important to understand how we are going to lose the weight. The three monosaccharides are:

1. **GLUCOSE**. This is the energy carb. It's found in fruits and vegetables. Eventually, all carbohydrates will be reduced to glucose through digestion.
2. **FRUCTOSE**. Also known as the fruit sugar. It's found in fruit, honey, and high-fructose corn syrup.
3. **GALACTOSE**. I want you to think of galactose as the milk sugar. It's less sweet than the others and found in milk.

If a word ends in "ose," it's sugar. These three sugars affect the body differently, so each one that you ingest will cause a different reaction. Now, there are many foods that are a mix of those three sugars when they bond together. The fancy term is disaccharides, and they look like this:

1. Sucrose = Glucose + Fructose
2. Lactose = Glucose + Galactose
3. Maltose = Glucose + Glucose

There's also something called polysaccharides, which are long-chain carbohydrates that are made up of smaller carbohydrates. Dietary fiber is an example of a polysaccharide. Remember that because we're going to circle back to fiber shortly.

So, we get that all carbohydrates are sugars, right? Now I want you to remember that all sugars are not created equal. Remember when I said glucose is needed to fuel the body? You might be thinking, "But Bob, if all carbohydrates are sugar, and these sugars are broken down into glucose, aren't all carbs good?" No. Glucose is what we want, and while it's true that fructose will be broken down into glucose eventually, it doesn't mean we want to ingest a bunch of high-fructose corn syrup. The reason lies in our digestive process.

When you put a carb in your mouth, your body immediately begins to process it. Like I said before, as soon as it goes in the mouth it begins to break down into glucose. So, what kind of carbs should we be eating? For the most part, we want the type of carbohydrates that take a while to digest. This seems backward, right? You would think you want fast digestion, but that's false. When it comes to carbs, the slower the digestion, the better. We want to eat the carbs that travel slowly through the body. Why? Processed carbs (bad ones) are super quick to digest. Most of these super-quick carbs lead to a spike in your insulin, causing your body to get completely off balance. Off balance is not good. In terms of digesting carbs, slow and steady wins the race. Good carbs are the tortoise, and bad carbs are the hare. This is why we only want to eat good carbs. The junk is going to get your system off balance, but the good carbs will give you a steady flow of energy over a longer period. Next time you buy those chewy fruit candies from the checkout counter, pay attention to what happens when you eat them. You get a little spike in energy when the sugars are digested, but this happens so fast that your body doesn't have time to level out, so you crash very quickly. We don't want to crash. There is an exception to this rule, fruit, and we'll get into that shortly. For now, I want you to remember that carbs are fuel, but it's important that you fill up on the right kind.

Without carbs, your body will not have the fuel it needs. If you've tried a low-carb diet, you probably have experienced low energy, or what many people refer to as the "carb flu." Your body gets confused when you remove its number-one energy source, and it begins to scramble to find a new way of sustaining itself. Your body is telling you that you are doing something unnatural. When I was doing the low-carb thing, I had days when I had zero energy. You might be wondering how someone can survive on a carb-free diet, and that's because the body will start to turn protein into carbs, and use fat as a main energy source to get what it needs. It's searching for a fuel source. The body is smart, smarter than you think. Which is why, when it wants balance, it's going to do whatever it needs to do to get that balance.

When the body gets off balance, crazy things start to happen when it tries to correct the problem. Carbs aren't just needed to give us energy, they are also used to break down fat. Without the right number of carbs, a by-product will enter the body. This by-product is known as ketones. When your body creates ketones, you run the risk of ketosis. I like to think of ketosis as the body's way of telling you something ain't right. Now, you may have heard of a diet that is quite literally called the Ketogenic Diet. It's for people who want their body to enter ketosis. Like many of the other low-carb diets, there can be great weight loss as a result. However, it comes at the price of the loss of good complex carbohydrates and a whole lot of other negatives. Urine sticks are even involved. Unless I'm pregnant, I don't want to be peeing on a stick. Ever talk to someone on the ketogenic diet? You can tell right away because their breath is often bad. One type of ketone that is produced is called acetone. Acetone comes out in the breath (and urine), and it smells rotten. I'm talking dragon-breath bad. The point is, the body will adapt to whatever we give it, but it's on us to give it the right stuff. We must listen to our bodies when they are telling us what they need and what they don't. I want us to use what the body was MEANT to use for fuel, and that includes carbohydrates and the right mix of nutrients.

Speaking of the right nutrients, remember that I mentioned fiber? If you grab some food from your cupboard and look on the nutrition label, you'll notice dietary fiber is listed right under "Total Carbohydrates." This isn't by accident. Fiber *is* a carbohydrate. And you know how I said we want carbs that break down slowly in the body? Fiber doesn't break down at all. It can't be turned into the glucose energy we need. Instead, it travels through the system all on its own, absorbing water along the way. This is why we get great poops when we eat lots of fiber. Not only will fiber get those bowels flowing, but it will slow down the digestion cycle, which is why we feel fuller for longer after eating high-fiber foods. The fuller we feel, the less inclined we are to eat the bad stuff, right? High-fiber foods will help you steer clear of the junk you eat when you're hungry.

"But Bob, what if I'm gluten-free? How can I eat carbs if I can't have gluten?" Okay, I've heard this a lot. I mean, a LOT. Nowadays, people are collecting food allergies like they're Pokémon. While there are quite a few people with allergies, there are lots of others that are crying wolf. The journal *Digestion* recently published a study that found that 86 percent of people who *believed* they were gluten-sensitive were actually gluten-tolerant.[2] That means quite a few people are buying gluten-free when they don't have to. My advice is always to go to the doctor and get an allergy test. It's completely possible you have a reaction to gluten, but you won't know it unless you get checked. If you are running around telling everyone you are allergic to gluten when you're not, you're doing your body more harm than good (and you're annoying your friends who may be allergic to gluten). If you think you are having a negative reaction when you are eating gluten, perhaps it's some-thing else. For me, if I don't have a protein and a fat with my carbs, I get . . . gassy. Sorry to gross you guys out, but it's the truth, and the truth can be hard to hear sometimes. I wasn't gassy because of the gluten, I was gassy because I wasn't properly combining my macros (macros=the grams of protein, carbs, and fat you consume). If you have a properly balanced meal, your insides will be properly balanced. I'm going to teach you how to do this in the next chap-ter, so stay tuned!

SUPER TIP: Aside from fuel and fiber, carbohydrates have a positive effect on the mood when partnered with the amino acid tryptophan. We usually only hear about trypto-phan during Thanksgiving when we use it as an excuse for why we take a few naps after eating turkey. Tryptophan is found in proteins, and in conjunction with carbohydrates, it increases serotonin, the stuff that makes you feel good. If you feel good, you're more likely to keep eating healthy and make it to the gym, right? A happy mind will lead to a happy body. Have I sold you on carbs yet?

If carbs don't make you fat, what does? Simple. Overeating. Your body needs carbs for energy, but when you eat too much, the excess is turned into fat. Your body needs a certain amount of every-thing, not just carbs, and when you eat more than you need, it be-comes fat. Sure, there are other factors, but the most basic and simple answer is that overeating is the primary cause of weight gain. The U.S. Department of Agriculture estimates that Americans eat 1,996 pounds of food per year. Not only that, but the *New York*

Times reported in 2010 that Americans consume 31 percent more packaged food than fresh food.[3] These numbers are TOO HIGH. Do our bodies need that much food? No. And they certainly don't need that much packaged food! If we don't need that much, why are people eating that much? I have a few theories. First, so many of our foods are filled with empty calories. That means food without any nutrients. Those carbs that digest superfast are entering and leaving the body at such a rapid rate that you're craving more and more. Nothing is filling. Everything is a large portion without sustenance. Second theory: ease. The crappy food is more readily available. It's much easier to grab some hot fries from the gas station than it is to stop at a grocery store when we are hungry. Even if the gas station has a few healthy options, it's more tempting to grab the KitKat from the checkout counter than it is the old banana. Finally, addiction. The wrong food can be addictive. We crave the bad stuff. It's made to be addictive. You don't think these large food corporations are stupid, do you? They know exactly what they're doing, and they're doing it well. We must be smarter than they are. The first step in being smarter? Knowing it's not the carbs that are making you fat.

SUPER TIP: Butter is not a carb. It's a fat. #Regina George

When I did the low-carb thing, my body eventually adjusted to the changes. The large amounts of protein I ate were used as carbs, just like we talked about, but the moment I had a real carb again, my body went into survival mode. I wasn't getting the balance I needed. Like I said before, the body is smart, so you won't be able to trick it for too long. If it wants a carb, it wants a carb. A no-carb lifestyle isn't sustainable. Many people like it for the fast results, but it always comes back to bite you in the butt in the end. I'm sure you've seen friends, family, or yourself lose weight quickly when cutting out the carbs, only to balloon up again as soon you had a slice of bread. We've all been there, even me. For a long time, I was a champion of the paleo diet, but ultimately I found its faults. My weight wasn't where I wanted it to be, and the results weren't worth what I was giving up. I still want you to get fast results, but I don't want you to run the risk of gaining it all back the minute you slip. That's why I created this plan.

Carbs can be tricky to understand. Complex, if you will. The scientific stuff can be confusing, but it's important to understand as you make the necessary changes in your diet. As we've learned, all carbs are not created equal. What I want you to remember most is that they do have a place in a well-rounded diet because the good carbs will fuel your body. The workouts at the end of this book will be possible by filling up your tank with the right kinds of nutrients. The right food will make it possible for you to lose weight and maintain the body you've always wanted. Remember, it's not carbs that are making you fat. It's overeating. I'm saying that so much because I want it to seep into your heads. We're changing the way you think, so you can change the way you look. Carbs don't make you fat. Carbs don't make you fat! CARBS DON'T MAKE YOU FAT! Okay, I think you get it. Now that we've changed the way we think, let's change the way we look.

2.

THE PLAN

MEN

Three square meals per day, plus one "floater" meal per day, for 90 days.

1. 160 calories from carbs per meal for three main meals.
2. 136 calories from protein per meal for four meals.
3. 135 calories from fat per meal for four meals.
4. 75 extra calories from vegetables per meal for three main meals.

*Based on men weighing 185 pounds and women weighing 135 pounds.

= 506 calories per meal for three main meals, plus 271 calories per floater meal, for a total of 1,789 calories per day.

WOMEN

Three square meals per day, plus one "floater" meal per day, for 90 days.

1. 120 calories from carbs per meal for three main meals.
2. 100 calories from protein per meal for four meals.
3. 108 calories from fat per meal for four meals.
4. 75 extra calories from vegetables per meal for three main meals.

    = 403 calories per meal for three main meals, plus 208 calories per floater meal, for a total of 1,417 calories per day.

EVERYONE

7–9 hours of sleep per night.

Weigh your food.

Weigh yourself.

Work out.

Monitor your waist.

THE MATH

Everyone is different, so everyone's numbers will be different, too. The above numbers are based on my own weight at 185 pounds. The women's column was calculated using a 135-pound woman. The numbers are in calories. I'm giving you the caloric numbers up front because I need you to understand why I am giving you all these numbers. Most people think in terms of calories when dieting. That's going to change when we convert to grams. You won't have to worry about conversion later, but for now we need to start with calories. First, I need you to pull out your calculator, or open the calculator app on your phone, and grab a pen and paper. We are going to get your numbers and personalize this plan for you. I know this part isn't fun. It's complicated, and I need you to know that's okay! It was complicated for me when I was figuring all this out. I get it. But if you want to take control of your life, I need you to put in some work. Ready? Let's break it down and get into how I got those numbers.

IMPORTANT

1 gram of carbohydrates = 4 calories

1 gram of protein = 4 calories

1 gram of fat = 9 calories

These numbers came from counting macronutrients. Maybe you've heard of this idea before. It's the process of keeping track of the grams of our three major nutrients, or macronutrients—carbs, protein, and fat. In some circles, there is a fourth "macronutrient" that is probably familiar to many of you, which is alcohol. We'll get into that later, but for now I want to focus on the main, real, macronutrients: carbs, protein, and fat.

There are three main meals on the Super Carb Diet, plus one "floater" meal. With each of the three main meals you can have carbs, protein, and fat. For the floater meal I don't want you having any carbs, just protein and fat. Let's start with the three main meals: breakfast, lunch, and dinner. I want men to be eating 40 grams of carbs per meal for the three main meals. For women, it's 30 grams. There are 4 calories in 1 gram of carbohydrates. Therefore, men should be having 160 calories from carbs per meal, and women no more than 120 calories from carbs per meal. Are you still with me? That's just one piece of the puzzle, so I want you to write down the number of calories from carbs on the paper in front of you.

Our protein and fat can be eaten at four meals. That's breakfast, lunch, dinner, and a fourth floater meal consisting of JUST the protein and fat. For the protein in every one of your four meals per day, you should be eating .75 grams of protein for every pound you weigh. For me, that's 139 grams of protein per day since I weigh 185 pounds ($185 \times .75 = 138.75$ grams, which rounds up to 139). This number is per day, so we need to divide it by 4 (the number of meals I want you eating per day). I know, I know, math is hard, right? It will all make sense soon, so just stick with me. Okay, where were we . . . 139 divided by 4 is 34.75, which I'm rounding DOWN to 34. Why am I rounding down to 34 here when the number is 34.75? Because I want to lose weight. That little bit is going to help. That's 34 GRAMS of protein per meal. Now we can convert the number into calories. Remember that there are 4 calories in 1 gram of protein, which means I take that 34 grams and multiply it by 4 to get the number of calories from protein per meal. The number comes out to 136. For me, that means 136 calories from protein per meal. To get your protein number:

1. Multiply your weight (in pounds) by .75.
2. Divide that number by 4.

That will give you the number of grams of protein you should be eating at each meal. Multiply the number of grams of protein for each meal by 4 to get the number of calories from protein per meal.

Write your number down.

Next is fat. There are 9 calories in 1 gram of fat. Men should be eating 15 grams of fat per meal. For women, it's 12 grams. If we multiply these numbers by 9 (because there's 9 calories in every gram of fat), it means men should have 135 calories from fat per meal, while women should be getting no more than 108 calories from fat.

Write that number down.

You see where these numbers are coming from, right?

1 gram of carbohydrates = 4 calories
1 gram of protein = 4 calories
1 gram of fat = 9 calories

It all circles back to those equivalents.

Finally, we have the vegetable number. Remember, for your three main meals you get to have some extra veggies ON TOP OF the carbs, protein, and fat. For EVERYONE, I want you to focus on getting 75 calories per meal strictly from vegetables for those three main meals. We'll talk more about those leafy greens in a bit, but for right now I want you to write down 75 for the calories from vegetables per meal.

You should have four numbers in front of you, all calories. If you add these up, you get the total number of calories PER meal that you should be eating. For me, at 185 pounds, that's 506 calories per each meal for breakfast, lunch, and dinner, plus 271 calories for that floater meal (which is JUST protein and fat), which gives me a total of 1,789 calories per day on the Super Carb Diet. Remember, these are caloric numbers.

I know I'm giving you a lot of numbers. Believe me, I felt like Russell Crowe in *A Beautiful Mind* trying to create the right equation for this program. Since it is so confusing at first, I want to go through it from a different angle. Here it is broken down even further:

BREAKFAST, LUNCH, AND DINNER

FOR MEN: 160 (calories from carbs) + the number of calories you got when you calculated your protein calories + 135 (calories from fat) + 75 (calories from vegetables) = the total number of calories per meal (for breakfast, lunch, and dinner).

FOR WOMEN: 120 (calories from carbs) + the number of calories you got when you calculated your protein calories + 108 (fat) + 75 (vegetables) = the total number of calories per meal (for breakfast, lunch, and dinner).

FLOATER MEAL

FOR MEN: The total number of calories you calculated for protein + 135 (calories from fat) = total calories in floater meal.

FOR WOMEN: The total number of calories you calculated for protein + 108 (calories from fat) = total calories in floater meal.

Now that we understand the calorie counts, how do we make sure we get the right amount of each for every meal? By counting the grams of carbs, protein, and fat in the food we put in our body.

For items with a nutrition label, this is easy. Grab anything out of your cupboard with a nutrition label on it. If you convert the grams using our handy formula, you'll notice they equal the number of calories listed on the label. Since you may have forgotten that formula, here it is again:

1 gram of carbohydrates=4 calories

1 gram of protein=4 calories

1 gram of fat=9 calories

I had some brown rice in my cupboard so I pulled out the box. The label looks like this:

Nutrition Facts Serving Size 1 Cup (125g) Servings Per Container 2 **Calories** 210 Calories from Fat 40	Amount/Serving	%DV*	Amount/Serving	%DV*
	Total Fat 3.5g	5%	**Potassium** 140mg	4%
	Sat. Fat 0g	0%	**Total Carb.** 40g	13%
	Trans Fat 0g		Fiber 2g	8%
	Cholest. 0mg	0%	Sugars 0g	
	Sodium 150mg	6%	**Protein** 5g	

*Percent Daily Values (DV) are based on a 2,000 calorie diet.

Iron 2% · Thiamin 15% · Niacin 15% · Folate 2%
Not a significant source of Vitamin A, Vitamin C, and Calcium.

INGREDIENTS: WATER, WHOLE GRAIN BROWN RICE, SUNFLOWER OIL, SALT, SOY LECITHIN.
CONTAINS: SOY

Listed here are 40 grams of carbs, 5 grams of protein, and 3.5 grams of fat. By using the equation above, I see that there are 160 calories from carbs (40×4), 20 calories from protein (5×4), and 31.5 calories from fat (3.5×9) in one serving. Those three numbers (160, 20, and 31.5) add up to equal the total number of calories listed (210, rounded). Now that we understand how to convert the grams to calories, we can use our scale to convert the food to fit our needs.

At the beginning of this chapter, I broke down the number of calories you should be eating at each meal. I did this because most of you are used to counting calories, but for this program we will need to just count the grams. If we're talking grams, I want you to create your plate this way:

MEN

Three main meals per day, plus one floater meal.

1. 40 grams of carbs per meal for **three** main meals (**none** for the floater).
2. 34 grams of protein per meal for **four** meals.
3. 15 grams of fat per meal for **four** meals.
4. 75 calories from vegetables for **three** main meals (**none** for the floater).

WOMEN

Three main meals per day, plus one floater meal.

1. 30 grams of carbs per meal for **three** main meals (**none** for the floater).
2. 25 grams of protein per meal for **four** meals.
3. 12 grams of fat per meal for **four** meals.
4. 75 calories from vegetables for **three** main meals (**none** for the floater).

You'll notice that these numbers line up with the calorie numbers once they are converted. The numbers are based on my weight at

185 pounds, and for women at 135 pounds. The protein numbers will change based on your current weight. So, you're asking, why don't we just count the total number of calories per meal and ignore the breakdown of carbohydrates, protein, and fat? Because each macronutrient has a very specific role to play in the body. If we simply follow a low-calorie diet without regard to which foods we're eating, we will compromise our body's functions, things like muscle loss and increased hunger, which we don't want to do when we are losing weight. Counting macronutrients is difficult at first, but once you get used to it you will see how easily it comes to you. You may be reading all these instructions and feel confused as all hell, but after the ninety days you will look back on these calculations and it will all make perfect sense.

I hope you survived all that math and got your numbers. Since you've made it this far, I should tell you I did the math for you at the end of this chapter. I gave you the numbers you need based on your weight. If you don't fall within the ranges I listed, you'll have to use that calculator app and get your numbers yourself. Now, I want you to remember that the numbers we calculated are the HIGH END of what I want you to be eating. That means you have to be flexible. If you aren't losing the weight you want to, adjust. As you lose the weight, your numbers will change. Your total number of calories per meal will decrease as your weight decreases because your protein needs are based on your current weight. When that happens, I need you to go back to the equation and update your calorie totals. That's why, among other reasons, I need you to be stepping on that scale to monitor your weight. There are a few other guidelines on this diet, so let's break this all down even more! You ready?

THE BREAKDOWN

First things first: three square meals per day, plus one *floater meal*. That means no snacks. You eat four times per day. That's it. I know that having a million small meals is all the rage, but not on my plan. I want you to have breakfast, lunch, and dinner, plus one meal that is going to essentially be your snack. I call it the floater meal. That means zero other snacks. Zero! The floater meal is your snack, and it's substantial. In lieu of snacking throughout the day, I am giving you the floater meal, which has the same amount of protein and fat as your three main meals but none of the carbs. Some athletes refer to this fourth meal as a second lunch, or second dinner, or maybe for you it will be what you are used to as a nighttime snack. The days are long, and sometimes three meals are just not enough. The floater meal is going to give you the option to have a protein bar after a workout, or some hearty food after dinner. That extra meal can come whenever you want. Just know that it is taking the place of all the snacks you usually eat throughout the day, and there are no carbs allowed with this meal. I know this is called the Super Carb Diet, but there must be limits.

If you're the type of person who has a bag of chips or popcorn every day, you'll have to get used to only eating four times a day. I tend to have my floater meal at night, after dinner. I get hungry before bed. You might, too. If you do, just plan that floater meal for the evening so you are eating something healthy instead of reaching for the pint of ice cream. I know you get hungry; believe me, I do. I'm working with you to make sure you never eat that pint of ice cream. I never, ever want you reaching for it, so that's why I'm giving you that extra meal. You shouldn't always need the floater meal, but it's there. You should be leaving breakfast, lunch, and dinner feeling fully satisfied because these meals have healthy portions. When I say fully satisfied after a meal, that doesn't mean STUFFED. There's a big difference between being satisfied and being too full. It's the difference between walking away from the dinner table and being rolled away from the dinner table. I want you to walk (or strut) away. I already said I'm going to get you to change the way you think, and here is a bridge to my next lesson—you don't need to feel full all the time. It's okay to be hungry. You shouldn't starve, but a little hunger is good.

People eat way more than they need to, and hardly anyone even has any idea how much they're eating these days. A Harvard Medical School study found that people surveyed at a variety of restaurants thought they were eating less than they were. Harvard's Jason Block wrote, "At least two thirds of all participants underestimated the calorie content of their meals, with about a quarter underestimating the calorie content by at least 500 calories."[1] That's more than an entire meal on the Super Carb Diet. It's a substantial amount. And what did we learn earlier? If you overeat, you're going to gain weight. That's why you need to know how much you're eating. Keeping it to three square meals per day (plus the floater meal) is going to make it easier to keep track of what goes into your body, and our food counting is going to keep you accountable.

Seems doable, right? And don't forget, I'm giving you carbs! It's all about turning your plate into a math equation. The way we're going to do that is by weighing our food. For the foods without the nutrition labels, you will need to get the measurements so you can track the calories in each meal. That means getting a food scale.

There's not a lot of equipment needed for the Super Carb Diet, but I am going to ask you to invest in a food scale and a body scale. I know a food scale can be daunting at first if you've never used one, but like everything else on this plan, it will be easier to use the longer you do it. Each time you are putting together your meal, just set your ingredients on the scale and measure them. What a hassle, right? It's important, though. Measuring your food will help you see what you're eating more clearly. Most people think they're eating light when they're really eating enough for two (or three or four). I see it all the time! If you take the time to weigh each thing that goes into your body, you will be much more conscious of the choices you are making and get a much stronger grasp on the quantity you put in your body. You can pull the food scale out before every meal, or you can meal-prep ahead of time to make things a little quicker. Clients always tell me that once they start using a food scale, they truly see how much they are eating. The numbers don't lie. A food scale will open your eyes to the truth on your plate. They sell them everywhere, and they are relatively inexpensive. Invest. They even make little travel scales you can throw in your purse or gym bag, so no excuses!

No matter how you weigh it, you're going to be cooking. I know, I know, you're thinking about how much time it is going to take to be cooking all these meals. You're right. It's going to take some time, but it's another investment in your future and an investment in your health. You got this book because you want to make a change, and change is not going to be easy. It's going to take time. If you're like Carrie Bradshaw and use your stove for storage, I want you to go clean it out right now because you're going to need it. Later, I'll share some recipes I use that make up a balanced Super Carb plate. In the meantime, I recommend planning your meals in advance, making grocery lists and so forth. And remember, this means no eating out. Nowadays some restaurants put the calories on the menu, and they will cater to every picky eater that walks in. Even so, I want you to try your best to stay away. Eventually, you'll have the tools you need to eat out, but for now, I want you to forget about restaurants. It's only ninety days out of your life. You can do it. There's too many unknown factors when you go out to eat, and you will be tempted to cheat. Not only that, but it's no fun to eat out with someone who is weighing their food when it comes to the table, so spare your friends. It's a pain in the butt, but your butt is going to look fantastic on the Super Carb Diet.

I also mentioned getting a body scale. Most people will tell you not to these days. I want you to. You should be seeing the numbers, not to obsess, but to understand. Weigh yourself every day to keep yourself accountable. As your weight goes down, the number of calories I want you ingesting will be going down, too, because that protein number is based on your current weight. It's not just important to weigh ourselves for the equation, it's also to help us monitor our progress. My best friend Cristi's mom, Joanne, is in her seventies. She's in fantastic health, and ever since I can remember she has maintained her weight. Her secret? She weighs herself every day. She'll tell you she wakes up each morning and hops on that scale. If she isn't within five pounds of the weight she is comfortable at, then she cuts back on her eating. She never fluctuates more than those five pounds because she knows the moment she starts to gain weight, she's accountable. Five pounds is a little drastic, so I recommend staying within ten pounds of that goal weight once you achieve it, but the idea is the same. Keep yourself accountable. On *The Biggest Loser,* we don't just weigh contestants because it makes for great TV. It also gives contestants a visual goal. The numbers will go up or down a few pounds if you're holding water or sweating a little bit more than usual, but I promise they will never fluctuate more than ten unless you've gained the actual weight. Ideally, you will weigh yourself when you wake up. Naked. And on a calibrated scale. Whatever time of day you decide to weigh yourself, just be sure it's the same time every single day. Consistency is key when it comes to the scale. I like the morning because you haven't consumed anything for the day and it will remind you of your goals for the day ahead.

Aside from stepping on a scale, I want you to measure your waist. Why? So you have another gauge for how you are doing. You may be losing body fat, but not body weight. If you keep track of your waist size, you'll get a better idea of what you need to alter based on your personal goals. For instance, those numbers we calculated earlier? They were all on the high end. Everybody is different. I cannot stress that enough. It is up to you to monitor your progress and adjust when necessary. Maybe you're finding that you're eating too much and not making any changes. If that's the case, you'll know when the scale-and-waist numbers are stagnant. When you start this program, I want you to get out a tape measure and measure the circumference of your waist in inches. To measure:

1. Remove your shirt.
2. Find your waist by gliding your fingers from the bottom of your rib cage to the top of your hips. Your waist will

be the soft section in between the two (usually the belly-button falls right in the middle of your waist).

3. Stand up straight and exhale.
4. Hold one end of the tape measure at your belly button and wrap the other end around your back until the two ends meet.

This number is your waist in inches. Write the number down on that piece of paper you have in front of you. Every week take out your tape measure and repeat the process. Monitor whether you are losing inches and adjust your numbers accordingly. Each body is different. I didn't want to just write a book with cookie-cutter answers on how to lose weight. I wanted to craft a plan that is unique to you, but that means you are going to have to do some of the work. Again, I know this isn't easy, but the accountability is going to ensure your progress.

Now let's circle back to that plate of food. I told you we're putting carbs back on it, and that's what I want you to think about first when you're making your food. I'm giving you 40 grams per meal (for your three main meals) if you're a man, and 30 grams per meal if you're a woman. That's a good number of carbs. Of course, it doesn't mean any ol' carb. It means the good stuff. There's carbs, and there's *carbage*. Next chapter I'll explain the difference.

After you get your carbs on your plate, I want you to find your protein number. That number will vary based on your weight, so be sure to pay attention to what you weigh when you calculate your exact protein number. It will end up being a good amount of meat, but it's not unlimited bacon like some of the other diets out there. I was vegetarian for a while, so I know a lot about the positives and negatives when it comes to eating meat. Immediately following my heart attack, I was completely vegetarian again. Then I slowly reintroduced other foods into my diet. There are so many wonderful benefits of being vegetarian. While this diet is not vegetarian, I want you to keep the red meat to a minimum. Ultimately, I crafted the Super Carb Diet protein quantities with that in mind. It will force you to keep the red-meat intake low. As a rule, even outside of this plan, I think that it's best to limit red meat to two to three times a month, at most, if you can.

Finally, I want men to have 15 grams of fat per meal, while women should have 12 grams per meal. It's a decent amount of fat, but again, the Super Carb Diet isn't a paleo diet. Your fats are going to be the oils you use in the kitchen plus some of the other foods that will expand the numbers on your plate. After my heart attack, I learned quite a bit about the Mediterranean diet and the wonderful benefits of healthy fats like olive oil. I used all that info to help formulate the fat contents of this diet.

The carbohydrates, protein, and fat are portioned out with weight loss and health in mind. I didn't just pick these numbers out of thin air. The meals are balanced. It's designed to help you lose weight while maintaining your heart health. And guess what? That's not all you get. For my athletes, or anyone looking to beef up their plate (no pun intended), you can have 75 calories of the leafy, green, cruciferous vegetables for breakfast, lunch, and dinner. In general, I want you to be sure you have an extra 75 calories of vegetables on your plate for each meal. No one has ever gotten fat eating broccoli unless it was covered in cheese, so please steam some greens and add them to your plate! The green vegetables are the ace in our pocket. They are going to round out each meal so that we are leaving satisfied. It's going to bulk up those other foods (just wait until you try my chicken and Brussels sprouts recipe) so your plate looks and tastes substantial.

Weighing and counting the foods to fit within the parameters of your numbers will be tricky at first. After you've been doing the Super Carb Diet for a while, you will be able to create your plate without looking at the scale. This is why we are doing it for ninety days. By the end of those ninety days, you will be accustomed to our equation. Until then, I want you following the numbers exactly. Your brain will start to form habits. You will instinctively know what makes a balanced meal by then without a food scale. It's just like riding a bike. At first, it will seem like a challenge, but once you get the hang of it, you will not think twice. I want you to get to the point where you can look down at your lunch and think, "I need more protein," or, "This doesn't seem like enough food, I should add some greens." While you're getting your bearings, you will constantly be checking food labels or using Google to tell you how many calories are in a bowl of oats. Eventually, the numbers will get easier.

The last piece of the Super Carb pie is sleep. I want you to do everything you can to get seven to nine hours of sleep each night. Every. Single. Night. The National Heart, Lung and Blood Institute recommends seven to eight hours of sleep per night.[2] I'm going with seven to nine because it varies for individuals and I want you well rested. This isn't just something that should be done as part of the Super Carb Diet. Sleep is the secret to success. If you don't sleep enough, you won't make good decisions. And I need you to make good decisions. It's going to be hard to eat that balanced meal when you can barely keep your eyes open. I want you to be alert, and I want your body to be ready for the changes you are making. Plus, I know how little you're all sleeping. There's Twitter, and Instagram, and Netflix & chill. These things are turning our beds into offices and we need more sleep. All of us. So please turn off the TVs and computers and get some shut-eye.

Those are my rules. Four meals per day. Carbs, protein, and fat for each of the three main meals. Protein and fat for the floater meal. Weigh your food. Weigh yourself. Measure your waist. Work out (more on that later!). Sleep. Simple, right? Plus, I gave you carbs! Coming up, I'll teach you the difference between good carbs and bad carbs so you can fill that plate up properly. After all, not all carbs are created equal.

P.S. I'm not just giving you carbs. I'm also giving you your numbers in a handy chart. These are the grams of carbs, protein, and fat you're allowed for all three main meals in a super-handy chart. Plus, don't forget you also get 75 calories from veggies for those three main meals. For the floater meal, you ONLY get the amount of protein and fat from the chart. And remember, I rounded DOWN with the protein numbers. Rounding down is going to help keep us slim. I still want you to know how to do the equation on your own, but just in case you need a little help:

MEN

Men's Weight (lbs.)	Grams of Carbs/Meal	Grams of Protein/Meal	Grams of Fat/Meal
180	40	33	15
185	40	34	15
190	40	35	15
195	40	36	15
200	40	37	15
205	40	38	15
210	40	39	15
215	40	40	15
220	40	41	15
225	40	42	15
230	40	43	15
235	40	44	15
240	40	45	15
245	40	45	15
250	40	46	15
255	40	47	15
260	40	48	15
265	40	49	15
270	40	50	15
275	40	51	15
280	40	52	15

WOMEN

Women's Weight (lbs.)	Grams of Carbs/Meal	Grams of Protein/Meal	Grams of Fat/Meal
130	30	24	12
135	30	25	12
140	30	26	12
145	30	27	12
150	30	28	12
155	30	29	12
160	30	30	12
165	30	30	12
170	30	31	12
175	30	32	12
180	30	33	12
185	30	34	12
190	30	35	12
195	30	36	12
200	30	37	12
205	30	38	12
210	30	39	12
215	30	40	12
220	30	41	12
225	30	42	12
230	30	43	12

3.

GOOD CARBS

Remember, all carbs aren't created equal. There are good carbs and there's "carbage." You're allowed 30 to 40 grams of carbohydrates per main meal on the Super Carb Diet, but that doesn't mean I want you loading up on potato chips. In fact, there should be no potato chips on your plate. Zero. And no pretzels. None. I want you to be focusing on carbs that will give you the energy you need and not processed junk.

What makes a carb a good carb? First and foremost, we want carbs that take a while to digest, remember? You already may have heard carbohydrates referred to as simple or complex. This all goes back to that rate of digestion we talked about earlier. The simple carbs are the hare, the super-quick sources of energy that are very rapidly digested. On the other hand, complex carbohydrates are the good ones, the tortoise. They are found in whole plant foods, are high in vitamins and minerals, and generally take a while to digest (good). They keep us full for longer because of the high fiber and long-lasting energy sources.

Simple carbs = Fast

Complex carbs = Slow

That doesn't mean ALL simple carbs are bad. Some, like fruit, are loaded with vitamins and minerals that are great for the body. Again, fruit is a simple carb, but it is not a BAD carb. I want to make sure you understand that not all simple carbs are created equal. For the most part, we want complex carbs, but fruit is the exception to the rule. The main difference between good carbs and carbage is added or unnatural sugar.

Think about bread for a minute. We all know that bread is a carb-heavy food. Most people hear "carb" and think "bread." Bread is certainly not the best carbohydrate on the market, but it tends to be the one people associate most with the word. When you're in the grocery store, there is a whole aisle filled with the stuff. If you're looking for carbohydrates, you can grab any old loaf of bread, right? No. That would be too easy. Next time you're in the bread aisle, look at the labels. You'll see white, wheat, rye, or whole grain. There's sandwich thins and mini bagels. Hawaiian rolls and brioche buns. If you're anything like me, you're salivating just thinking about all the choices. However, if you start to look at the labels, you'll quickly lose your appetite. That's because many of these are the bad, simple carbohydrates. They are loaded with sugars (not the naturally occurring sugar you get with fruit) and additives, the stuff that will keep you from getting to your goal weight. They will go in your body and satisfy you for a few brief moments until you're hungry for something else. There are, however, some bread options that *will* fill you up. I'm talking about the 100 percent whole-grain bread. Usually, it's the loaf with the soonest expiration date. That may be inconvenient for those of us who don't want to go to the store a hundred times a month, but it is good for our bodies. Keep in mind that you shouldn't eat a whole loaf, but if it fits into your plate equation, then you can eat the good stuff. Fresh bread, with little preservatives or additives, is what you want to look for. Stay away from white bread. No good comes from white bread. Every time you see white bread I want you to think of me. Picture me telling you to run away from it. Imagine the white bread is covered in flames and you are unable to even pick it up. White bread is my arch-nemesis, the Joker to my Batman. The Saruman to my Gandalf. The Joan to my Christina.

Okay, so now we all understand bread, but what about all the other good carbs? In general, the same theory applies: know what you're buying and what you're eating. Are you looking at the nutrition labels every time you shop? We want foods without *any* added sugars. Caloric sweeteners, high-fructose corn syrup, and other syrups are terrible for you. If you look at the ingredient label and see them, I want you to stay away. The best way to differentiate the good carbs from the carbage is to study the nutrition label before you buy a product.

When I'm grocery shopping, I *always* look at labels. As soon as you pick up a food, I want you to do the same. Don't get distracted by the cartoon characters on the package. I don't care about the branding on food, I want to know exactly what is in it. This is easy to do, but you need to grab the item and turn it over to get the facts. The bells and whistles on a package are there to distract you! Nutrition labels are on food for a reason. They aren't just there for decoration. If that were the case, I'd imagine they would be colorful and have cute little emojis next to each column. Instead, labels are in black and white with a basic and clear font so we can read them. Outside of those little black-and-white boxes you'll see buzzwords like "natural" or "healthy." These are distractions! Don't fall for them. They're buzzwords, almost always there to get you to buy something. Food packaging is purposely misleading to sell product.

The only thing I need to look at when I'm shopping for food is the nutrition label. On it you'll see the ingredients, and the total number of carbs, protein, and fat. It may take you some time to read all these labels at the store, so plan accordingly. We've all got a lot packed into our days, but I need you to set aside some extra time for your grocery shopping on the Super Carb Diet so you can read the labels. If you're pressed for time, avoid shopping on Saturdays. Jack Goodman of the Time Use Institute found that Saturday is the busiest day for grocery shopping, while Monday and Tuesday tend to be the least busy.[1] Use this information to your advantage. Plan ahead.

I've found in all my years of working with people who are trying to lose weight that so many don't understand how to read the labels. People are great at reading the prices on packaging, but they don't realize that the ingredient labels are what will save you money down the line. That's because even though some of these foods may be cheaper than the healthy stuff, they will cost more in the long run when you're running to the doctor. Of course, the company can't advertise the doctor bills that come later. Companies wouldn't stay in business if they wrote, "This will make you obese" on the box, would they? Sure, you can save a few pennies now by ignoring the nutrition label, but you can save *thousands* by reading it and bypassing those hospital bills for treating your deteriorating health. All the time people tell me that they can't eat healthy because it's too expensive. Yes, it *seems* like eating unhealthy will save you money. It won't. Your body will eventually shut down if you fill it with crap. Have you been to the doctor lately? It's expensive! Visits and prescriptions cost an arm and a leg. The more crap you eat, the more you will be scheduling appointments. Believe me, it's cheaper to eat healthy.

Let's get back to the nutrition labels, shall we? If you're reading this near your kitchen, grab something with a food label on it. First thing I want you to pay attention to is the serving size. I can't emphasize enough how important the serving size is. The Super Carb Diet will make your understanding of quantity so much better than before because you will be weighing your foods and counting the macronutrients to see exactly what you're eating. When it comes to packaged food, you need to look at that serving size even before you start to count those carbs, protein, fat, and veggies. Your eyes should immediately turn to that serving size when you pick up a packaged food. Don't get suckered into eating more or less than you think you are because you're ignoring the serving size. Before you do anything else, look at that serving size and think about how much you are putting on your plate and if it matches up to your calculated number. If it doesn't, adjust the numbers or adjust your plate. Don't ignore it. Serving size. Serving size! SERVING SIZE!

When it comes to carbs on the nutrition facts, you'll notice there is a "Total Carbohydrates" percentage along with a number in grams, and underneath that you'll see numbers for dietary fiber and sugar. The percentage is in relation to your entire daily diet, as recommended by the FDA. However, right now I want you to look at the label you have in front of you and focus on both the total grams of carbohydrates *and* the grams of dietary fiber and sugar. The total grams are what we are using to get those 30 to 40 grams of carbs per meal, remember? The grams in dietary fiber and sugar are going to tell us if these are good carbs or bad carbs. If the number of grams in the sugar column is high, it's no good for this diet. Make sense?

There are some exceptions. A food might have 15 grams of sugar listed, but it may be naturally occurring. Most fruits are high in sugar, and they are considered simple carbohydrates, but they are not carbage. Again, fruit is good! I don't want all this info to mislead you into thinking fruit is the devil. Because of the protein, fiber, and other nutrients in fruit, they act more like complex carbohydrates in the body. That certainly doesn't mean you should be eating barrels of oranges, but fruit in moderation is great. Plus, those of you that have a sweet tooth will need it to satisfy your cravings.

So, all fruit is good, right? Not so fast. Dried fruit comes packaged with nutrition labels, and if you look at the label, the sugar content is usually high. But it's just fruit, right? Not always. If the nutrition facts say there is lots of sugar, I want you to circle back to the ingredient list. Dried fruit can vary, depending on the company making it. Sometimes it will simply be the dried version of the fruit alone. Other times there will be added sugars and preservatives.

That's why I want you looking at the ingredient list. Always. I am NOT a fan of dried fruit. I find it to be very misleading. It's one of those foods everyone thinks is healthy, but I want you to stay away from it. Not only can the ingredients be deceiving, but it's something you think you are eating less of than you are. It's shrunk down so much that you end up eating way more sugar than you realize. You can eat the equivalent of six mangos as a snack because it just feels like a few bites. I feel similarly about nuts. Packaged nuts can have lots of additives, and most people eat more than a few. Fortunately, it's a bit easier to visualize what you're getting with nuts. With these foods and more, you need to get used to knowing exactly how much you are putting into your body. If you are going to eat them, be sure you aren't eating the wrong kind or more than the serving size. Check the labels! The ingredient list on a package of dried fruit or nuts could be one item, or it could be fifteen. Within those fifteen items, the quantity of each could vary.

Many people don't know this, but the ingredients are listed in order of quantity. If you see sweeteners or syrups listed in the first few ingredients, then I want you to put the food down and move on to something else because that means there are higher quantities of sweeteners or syrups than the ingredients that follow it. If there are five or more ingredients, regardless of what they are, chances are you can move on. It's carbage. Lengthy ingredient labels are a telltale sign that the food is no good for you. Read the nutrition labels!

Up until now, it might seem like finding the good carbs is going to be all about the packaging and studying the labels. Well, what about all those foods at the grocery store without any packaging? Ah, that's where you'll find the really, really good carbs. That's where you'll find them 99 percent of the time. It's because the whole foods are found in the perimeter of the grocery store. These are the fruits, vegetables, and nuts that are sold by the pound. In a perfect world, you would do all your shopping in the perimeter of a grocery store. I would love it even more if you did all your shopping at a farmers market. I take that back, I would be MOST happy if you had a garden and grew your own food. That's the best way to ensure that you are eating the very best. Since we don't all have the time for gardening, the grocery store will have to do. The point is, the perimeter is where you find all the fresh produce that is super flavorful and good for your system.

When you're shopping in the produce section, I want you to start looking at all the plant-based foods with lots of colors. These are the good carbs—the beautiful orange sweet potatoes, the rich blueberries, and the perfectly imperfect black-eyed peas. If you follow me on Instagram, you know I love photography. Every time I walk into a grocery store, I think about how beautiful the produce section is. The processed stuff has executives and artists carefully constructing every font and box, but the food inside the box often looks like crap. The produce, however, is beautiful. If I take my camera into the grocery store, I will head straight for the deep green vegetables and colorful fruits. Those pretty, whole foods are going to get you more "likes" any day of the week.

So, what *exactly* are the good carbohydrates I want you to eat on the Super Carb Diet?

WHOLE GRAINS. Whole grains have gotten a bad rap. People are scared to eat them. The truth is, 100 percent whole grains are wonderful. I'm here to take away the taboo. They are filled with fiber, which is going to aid in digestion and keep the poops running smoothly, as well as nutrients like iron, an essential mineral. Plus, we know that the fiber is going to keep us fuller, longer. Whole grains also help prevent chronic diseases. In 2011, the American Society for Nutrition found that whole grains reduce the risk of diseases like coronary heart disease, diabetes, and cancer.[2] I want you all to stop fearing whole grains and start embracing them as a part of the Super Carb Diet. With all that said, it's not just any grain you need. I want you to pay close attention to the grains you are buying. Just because something says "Whole Grain" on the packaging doesn't mean it's good for us. There's a difference between something labeled "Whole Grain" and something labeled "100% Whole Grain." We want the "100% Whole Grain" or the "100% Whole Wheat." If it isn't 100 percent, it means it's been stripped of a lot of the nutrients. More than that, we want to be certain it doesn't have a whole bunch of other ingredients in it. Steer clear of absolutely anything with high-fructose corn syrup. I said it before, but it bears repeating: stay away from products with lots of syrups or preservatives. Read the labels. I know I'm harping on this, but it's SO important. It's also one of the most common problems I see when I'm working with my clients. If you want to lose weight, you need to know what you're putting in your body. The only way to know is if you read the labels.

BEST SUPER CARB GRAINS

- Barley
- Brown rice
- Brown rice pasta
- Buckwheat
- Bulgur
- Couscous
- Farina
- Freekeh
- Gram flour
- Kamut
- Millet
- Montina flour
- Oatmeal
- Orzo
- Popcorn (air popped)
- Quinoa pasta
- Rye
- Semolina
- Sorghum
- Spelt
- Teff
- Tortillas (100% whole grain or 100% whole wheat)
- 100% Whole wheat bread
- 100% Whole wheat pasta
- 100% Whole wheat pita
- Wild rice

FRUITS. Fruits are high in sugar. There's no way around that. Granted, it's the good, naturally occurring sugar, but it's sugar nonetheless. When you're trying to lose weight, it's best to stay away from foods with such high amounts of sugar, even the good kind. Because we did the math earlier and figured out the number of calories and carbs you're allotted per meal, I think you'll find that you aren't reaching for fruit as much as you thought you would be. That's not to say there aren't fantastic low-carb fruits that fit into our plate equation. Fruits like raspberries and watermelon tend to be lower in carbs than apples, so they will work better with your numbers. If you opt for fruit, just be mindful of those digits. And know that if you are having a plate of blueberries, you aren't going to have room for that whole-grain bread. It's one or the other. Think about what foods you want to fill your plate up with. If you are craving sweets and worry you'll fall off the wagon without some chocolate, then have an orange instead of the brown rice. Make smart choices.

SUPER CARB FRUITS

- Apples
- Apricots
- Bananas
- Blackberries
- Blueberries
- Boysenberries
- Cantaloupe
- Cherries
- Cranberries
- Damson
- Dragon fruit
- Fig
- Grapes
- Grapefruit
- Goji berries
- Guava
- Honeyberry
- Honeydew
- Juniper berries
- Kumquats
- Lemons
- Limes
- Loquats
- Lychee
- Mangos
- Nectarines
- Oranges
- Peaches
- Plums
- Raspberries
- Strawberries
- Watermelon

VEGETABLES. I said it before, and I'll say it again: no one has ever gotten fat eating broccoli. You can eat it raw, grilled, roasted (my favorite), boiled, or sautéed. Throw it in your salad or rice bowl. Dip it in hummus or tahini. There are so many ways to eat broccoli and other vegetables, so fill up that plate with them. Vegetables are high in nutrients like vitamins A and C, folic acid, and potassium. I cannot recommend them enough! I want you to start thinking of vegetables in two different categories: leafy greens, and everything else. Leafy greens are a GREAT way to build your plate so you are feeling full and satisfied. Again, that doesn't mean lettuce covered in ranch dressing; that means just the lettuce. If it's a leafy green (without any oil or seasoning on it), it's Super Carb approved. Thinking of leafy greens in a separate category from your other vegetables is going to help train your brain to start adding them to *every* meal. Not only that, but on the Super Carb Diet, I give you 75 *extra* calories just for vegetables for those three main meals. If it's listed below, you're allowed 75 calories on top of the rest of your plate equation. That's because you should be eating more veggies. Everyone should. The more veggies you eat, the less crap you'll eat. Fill up on the good stuff and there won't be room for carbage.

SUPER CARB LEAFY GREENS

- Arugula
- Cabbage
- Chard
- Chinese cabbage
- Collard greens
- Curly endive
- Dandelion
- Garden cress
- Iceberg lettuce
- Kale
- Komatsuna (Japanese mustard spinach)
- Mâche
- Mizuna
- Mustard greens
- Romaine
- Spinach
- Tatsoi
- Watercress

SUPER CARB VEGGIES

- Artichokes
- Asparagus
- Beets
- Bell peppers
- Bok choy
- Broccoli
- Broccoflower
- Broccoli romanesco
- Brussels sprouts
- Butternut squash
- Carrots
- Cauliflower
- Cucumbers
- Daikon
- Eggplant
- Ethiopian mustard (also known as Ethiopian kale)
- Fennel
- Garlic
- Green beans
- Horseradish
- Jicama
- Kohlrabi
- Leeks
- Mushrooms
- Onions
- Parsnips
- Pumpkin
- Radishes
- Rutabaga
- Scallions
- Tomatoes
- Turnips
- Wild broccoli
- Yams
- Yellow summer squash
- Zucchini

BEANS/LEGUMES. Beans and legumes are filled with fiber, which is going to make you feel fuller longer. When I was a vegetarian, beans and legumes were my best friend. Sometimes people think beans are more of a protein, but they are loaded with carbs, so it's important to make note and not overindulge. The bean/legume category is also the one that most people ignore at the grocery store. If you find yourself leaving your lunch or dinner hungry, I want you to start filling your plate with a little more of these carbs.

SUPER CARB BEANS AND LEGUMES

- Adzuki beans
- Black beans
- Black turtle beans
- Chickpeas
- Cowpeas
- Cranberry beans
- Hummus
- Hyacinth beans
- Fava beans
- Great northern beans
- Kidney beans
- Lentils
- Lima beans
- Lupin beans
- Miso
- Mung beans
- Navy beans
- Pigeon peas
- Pink beans
- Pinto beans
- Tempeh
- Tofu
- Soybeans
- Split peas
- White beans
- Yellow beans

DAIRY. Dairy products tend to be high in carbs and fat, so you won't be filling up your plate with *too* much of them. I personally find that dairy causes a lot of extra mucus in my system, so I mostly stay away from it. I know people like their dairy, so I'm not here to take that away from you entirely. I just want to recommend the good stuff. If you want to put some milk in your coffee because you absolutely cannot drink it black, and you don't like almond milk, go with skim. As always, you'll have to factor it into your numbers. If you add that creamer (which is typically loaded with additives) to your coffee, that's going to mean less food on your plate. I also love my nonfat Greek yogurt for breakfast. You don't have to worry about high fat content, and you can jazz it up with some peanut butter, nuts, or seeds (just be mindful of how many nuts you are eating!). In terms of cheeses, I like cottage and feta best because they are low in fat, and Swiss because it contains a lot of phosphorous. Parmesan is also low in calories (in terms of cheese), and the robust flavor means a little bit goes a long way.

SUPER CARB DAIRY

- Cottage cheese
- Feta cheese
- Nonfat Greek yogurt
- Parmesan cheese
- Skim milk
- Swiss cheese

If you focus on the carbs that are directly from the earth, which can be grown in a garden, you'll be in good shape. Stick to plant-based foods without a lot of ingredients and you will find it easy to craft the perfect Super Carb plate. The main thing I want you to remember is that all carbs are not created equal. There's good carbs like the 100 percent whole grains, fruits, vegetables, beans, and legumes that I listed, and there's carbage. Next time you're at the grocery store, grab a cartful of the good carbs, and leave the carbage in Aisle 7.

4.

CARBAGE

Now that you know what the good carbs are, it's time for you to understand *carbage*. Carbage is the garbage. It's the stuff you put in your belly without caution. The problem is, most people don't even know when something is bad. Until now. Carbage is the carbohydrate-heavy processed foods that are absorbed quickly. Remember, slow and steady wins the race when it comes to carb digestion, and carbage is fast as hell.

We need to understand what happens when you eat carbs to understand the difference between the good carbs and carbage. When bad carbs enter the system, the blood sugar levels spike. Carbs are the main source of energy, so all carbs are going to give you energy when they enter your body. The carbs turn into glucose (sugar=glucose), and the sugar enters the bloodstream practically when you put it in your mouth. The problem is, sugar doesn't just immediately become energy when it gets into your system. That would be too easy. This is where insulin comes into play. The pancreas is what produces insulin, a hormone. Remember that: the pancreas produces insulin. Insulin is needed to do one of two things: use the sugar for energy, or store it for future use. Without insulin, the sugar is in the bloodstream, but it's useless. Insulin is what guides the sugar to the appropriate place, either to be stored as energy or used as energy.

Insulin can be quite confusing. I get it. Unless you've struggled with diabetes, it tends to be one of those words that you hear all the time but don't truly understand. I fly a lot, and I recently got to thinking about how insulin is like the flight attendants on a plane. When you board a plane, there are usually a few flight attendants guiding passengers to their seats. Without the attendants working diligently, the boarding gets backed up. Not only that, but if there are too many crew members performing this task, the aisle gets crowded and unruly. We've all seen this, right? It's a nightmare. Flying is already stressful without the disarray. If the crew isn't helping people get their luggage to the overhead bins and quickly to their seats, everything becomes chaos. Insulin is the flight attendant. Insulin guides the glucose to their seats for a smooth flight. When you eat good carbs, the sugar will process slowly but surely, keeping your blood sugar levels at a steady pace and make your body run as efficiently as possible. It's the perfect mix of efficient flight attendants and a manageable crowd of passengers. When the body gets carbage, the blood sugar levels spike rapidly, causing chaos. The usual amount of insulin is not equipped to handle the sudden rush, so the pancreas struggles to keep up. The aisle of the plane becomes a hot mess. It's the body's way of telling you that it does not know how to properly process those types of foods. Blood cells cannot handle the extra sugar and they will get damaged. This leads to type 2 diabetes and trouble.

By trouble, I mean sugar addiction. It is real. Extra insulin that is produced to handle a quick rush of sugar in the bloodstream will cause a sudden burst of energy. We all feel this happen when we eat a bag of candy. It's that quick sugar rush followed by a lull. The lull comes because so much extra insulin was produced to keep up with the blood sugar that now there is not enough blood sugar to keep up with the insulin. This causes the body to crave more. That's how it starts. The body is asking for more of that quick-fix sugar. I don't know about you, but this sounds like a surefire way for someone to get addicted to those quick-fix sugars. We don't want that. Extra sugar means extra pounds on your body. Not only do I want to ensure that you don't get a sugar addiction, I want to make sure you break the sugar addiction you may already be suffering from. The Super Carb Diet is going to reset everything. If you're in that cycle of getting your energy from those simple sugars, you're in for a surprise. And not a good one. It will take some time for your body to adjust. You will crave foods that will give you a quick jolt. This is undeniable. I can't help you in one of those moments, other than to tell you that it will pass. You must be strong. You must resist the temptation to reach for another candy bar. Don't do it. Wait for the moment to pass. Eventually, the body will remember its purpose and you will make it through the candy storm.

It's not just sugar addiction you need to worry about. It's type 2 diabetes. Type 2 diabetes develops because the insulin that is supposed to carry the glucose into storage for energy stops working.

The World Health Organization concludes that the number of people living with diabetes has increased from 108 million in 1980 to 422 million in 2014.[1] The numbers are rising. If you have type 2 diabetes, you must keep the level of glucose in your body within a healthy range. Diabetics should consult their doctor first to design a diet plan that is right for them. All that math we just did is going to save you from weekly doctor visits down the road, remember? I know this diet is hard. It's supposed to be. But it's going to save your life. You need to take it seriously because a poor diet is going to lead to things like diabetes and heart failure. We're so focused on looks, but there's a lot at risk besides your pants fitting properly. The carbage that goes into your body is actively destroying it. Stop it before it stops you.

I wrote a book called *Skinny Habits*. In it I give away the secrets of how people get and stay thin. One of the things I talk about is dressing for thinness. Of course, when you read that, you probably immediately think I'm concerned about vanity and nothing else. That couldn't be further from the truth. Looking great is going to make you feel great. The fact is, most of you are starting this diet because you want to look a certain way. Most people tell me they want to lose weight because they want to look good for their wedding, their prom, or a class reunion. Giving up carbage is hard, and losing weight for vanity is, in my experience, the best motivator. It gets people started, and once they start, their health follows. If looks are what it takes to get you started, then grab that mirror and get to staring. Come for the looks, stay for the health. It's why I do what I do. I want everyone to be healthy, and I want your bodies to endure.

The silver lining is that we do have some control over how we treat the body. We can choose to fill ourselves with the good carbs that will keep our engines running properly. That means no carbage. Stay away from all refined sugars. A good rule of thumb is to not eat anything with added sugar. Search for the foods with no labels in the perimeter of the grocery store. If you are buying something with a label, I want you to immediately look at that ingredient list. If there is sugar in the ingredients, set it down and walk away. Added sugar is going to ruin your body. Also, stay away from the corn syrups and sweeteners that have fancy names you can't pronounce. Say no to white bread, soda, candy, pretzels, chips (this one is hard for me), cake, anything with high-fructose corn syrup, cookies, or jams. If it's processed, it's probably a no from me. If it has *added* sugar, it's a definite no from me.

You are probably looking at most of those items and thinking, "No shit, Bob, of course I should stay away from cake on a diet." You're right, no shit. But there are some gray areas that may not be so clear. I'm talking about the fruits and the dairy, foods that are seemingly whole and good for us but don't contain the complex carbs I talked about earlier. In case it wasn't clear before, simple carbs aren't always bad, as long as the sugar is naturally occurring. The body will treat these simple carbs accordingly because the body is smart! While these carbs aren't carbage, they also won't help you lose weight if you eat large quantities. Moderation is key. Will a glass of milk make you obese and send you into a sugar addiction? Of course not. Does it have a place on your Super Carb plate? Yes and no. It's why we have our equations. Yes, you can have fruit and dairy. In moderation. I told you earlier I love a nonfat Greek yogurt in the morning. But remember, you have a specific number of carbs you are allowed, so an apple may not be the best use of that space on your plate. These foods are high in carbs, so if you want a banana at lunch, you can't have that brown rice. Plan accordingly.

Be wary of what you are putting into your body when it comes to fruit and dairy, like that dried fruit we discussed with the extra ingredients. And that's not all. Time and time again, I see people drinking juice and thinking it's fresh. Often it is from concentrate or even a juice "cocktail." These are no-nos. They're carbage. The same goes for dairy. Coffee creamer is not skim milk, and all yogurt is not created equal. You must look at the labels to see if there is *added* sugar. If there is, it's a no. Just because something is near other healthy foods in the grocery store, or just because it's labeled with buzzwords like "fat-free" or "healthy" does not mean it is good for you. Make certain you are getting fresh fruit and pure dairy if you are adding it to your plate; otherwise, you will risk getting right back into that sugar cycle. Take out the carbage, and you will be setting yourself up for long-term success. In case you aren't quite sure, I've made a list you can look at any time you need a reminder. These are the biggest carbage culprits that should not be getting a ride in your grocery cart any time soon.

CARBAGE

- Bagels
- Barbecue sauce
- Beer
- Bread sticks
- Cake
- Candy
- Cereal
- Cookies
- Corn
- Corn chips
- Corn nuts
- Corn syrup
- Crackers
- Cream of Wheat
- Donuts
- Dried fruit
- French fries
- Fried food
- Fruit cocktail
- Fruit juice
- Full-fat dairy
- Gummies

- Honey
- Honey-roasted nuts
- Ice cream
- Jam
- Jelly
- Juice cocktail
- Ketchup
- Maple syrup
- Margarine
- Muffins
- Pancakes (exception: my Protein Pancakes recipe on page 253)
- Pizza dough
- Popcorn (movie theater)
- Potato chips
- Pretzels
- Refined sugar
- Rice cakes
- Soda
- Smoothies (I'm not talking about your Super Carb protein shakes)
- Sweet tea
- Sweetened beverages
- Sweetened nut butters
- Sweetened yogurt
- Syrup
- Waffles
- WHITE BREAD
- White flour
- White pasta

5.

ALL ABOUT PROTEIN

You didn't think we would *only* talk about carbs, did you? There are two other macronutrients for which we've barely scratched the surface, and I need you to know about *everything* you're putting into your body. That means understanding protein and how we're going to make it work for you. I like to think of protein as the fertilizer in your garden. For those of you that want those big, lean muscles, you need to eat your protein. That is what's going to make your body grow (in the good way). Protein will work hand in hand with your time in the gym to help get your body where you want it to be. But before we get into all the ways protein works for us, we should recap the numbers:

Men's Weight (lbs.)	Grams of Protein/Meal	Women's Weight (lbs.)	Grams of Protein/Meal
180	33	130	24
185	34	135	25
190	35	140	26
195	36	145	27
200	37	150	28
205	38	155	29
210	39	160	30
215	40	165	30
220	41	170	31
225	42	175	32
230	43	180	33
235	44	185	34
240	45	190	35
245	45	195	36
250	46	200	37
255	47	205	38
260	48	210	39
265	49	215	40
270	50	220	41
275	51	225	42
280	52	230	43

MEN

Men's Weight (lbs.)	Grams of Carbs/Meal	Grams of Protein/Meal	Grams of Fat/Meal
180	40	33	15
185	40	34	15
190	40	35	15
195	40	36	15
200	40	37	15
205	40	38	15
210	40	39	15
215	40	40	15
220	40	41	15
225	40	42	15
230	40	43	15
235	40	44	15
240	40	45	15
245	40	45	15
250	40	46	15
255	40	47	15
260	40	48	15
265	40	49	15
270	40	50	15
275	40	51	15
280	40	52	15

WOMEN

Women's Weight (lbs.)	Grams of Carbs/Meal	Grams of Protein/Meal	Grams of Fat/Meal
130	30	24	12
135	30	25	12
140	30	26	12
145	30	27	12
150	30	28	12
155	30	29	12
160	30	30	12
165	30	30	12
170	30	31	12
175	30	32	12
180	30	33	12
185	30	34	12
190	30	35	12
195	30	36	12
200	30	37	12
205	30	38	12
210	30	39	12
215	30	40	12
220	30	41	12
225	30	42	12
230	30	43	12

Here are the numbers to stick to in terms of protein on the Super Carb Diet: .75 grams of protein per pound of your body weight, per day. We know there are 4 calories per gram of protein, so for me at 185 pounds, that's 136 calories (34 grams) from protein per meal for four meals (our three main meals AND our fourth floater meal). Right off the bat you'll notice something: these numbers are high. This is the cap, the numbers I don't want you going over. That's why I rounded down when I was calculating them. Can you have less? Yes. Can you have more? Absolutely not. This amount of protein is more than substantial. In fact, you will probably have a hard time reaching these levels of protein when you first start out. The biggest challenge will come from finding lean proteins without a lot of fat. Don't forget, we still need to stay within our carb-and-fat parameters, so you can't just load up on any meat to build up to your protein numbers. That would be too easy. Instead, you'll have to focus on the lean proteins that are low in fat. I'm talking poultry, egg whites, fish, bison, and pork.

I said I want you to be aware of everything you are putting into your body, which means you need to understand what protein is. And it's not just meat. Yes, there is a lot of protein in meat, but it's much more complex than that. Protein is part of every single cell in your body. You need it to build and repair tissues, and to make hormones and other chemicals in the body. It is 100 percent essential to life. For those of you keeping track at home, two things I absolutely, without a doubt, cannot live without: protein and Madonna's *Like a Prayer* album. (Could you imagine not being able to listen to "Express Yourself" during a workout? I'm not interested in living in a world without it.) Back to protein! Without any protein, your body simply won't work. Your body is the garden, and protein is the fertilizer.

Of course, you wouldn't have protein without amino acids because proteins are molecules that consist of amino acids. Amino acids attach to one another to form the proteins, and there are twenty of them. Within those twenty, there are two types:

1. Essential amino acids
2. Nonessential amino acids
   a. Conditional

Essential amino acids are the ones we get from food. Your body doesn't make these acids, so you need to get them elsewhere. There are nine of them for adults. Nonessential amino acids are still important, but they are considered nonessential because the body makes them. You see that little "a" under nonessential amino acids? Within this type, eight are considered "conditional" and three are not considered conditional. Still with me? What conditional means in this case is that your body produces them, but when you are sick or under a lot of stress, your body may not be producing *enough* of them for what you need, in which case you would benefit from adding them to your diet. Reports vary slightly on which amino acids are conditionally essential, but I've found that generally the eight marked below are considered conditional. Let's have a look.

ESSENTIAL AMINO ACIDS
1. Histidine
2. Isoleucine
3. Leucine
4. Lysine
5. Methionine

6. Phenylalanine
7. Threonine
8. Tryptophan
9. Valine

NONESSENTIAL AMINO ACIDS

1. Arginine (Conditional)
2. Tyrosine (Conditional)
3. Cysteine (Conditional)
4. Proline (Conditional)
5. Glutamine (Conditional)
6. Ornithine (Conditional)
7. Serine (Conditional)
8. Glycine (Conditional)
9. Alanine
10. Asparagine
11. Aspartate

Each of the amino acids serves a purpose in the body, but it's most important to focus on the essential amino acids in regard to our diet and eating habits. Some of these may be new to you, while some of you may know these amino acids best as supplements. If you head over to a vitamin and supplement store, you'll see these amino acids sold in pill or powder form. Since each amino acid serves a different purpose in the body, many people will supplement their diet if they are lacking in one or more of the essentials. We'll talk more about supplements and micronutrients later. In the meantime, isn't it best to get all you need from the food you are eating? The best sources of protein in food contain all nine of those essential amino acids. Remember how we wanted to focus on good carbs and weed out the carbage? Protein is similar. We want proteins with the nutrients we need most so that we are setting our bodies up to be as successful as possible. That means finding foods that are *complete protein sources*, the ones that contain all nine of the essential amino acids. What foods contain all nine?

1. **ANIMAL MEATS.** Animal meats are considered complete proteins. However, we have some numbers to keep track of. This means that many animal meats are going to be too high in fat to fit onto our plate equation. They still contain all nine amino acids, but they aren't going to work on the Super Carb Diet. There are, however, lots of great lean animal meats that give you all the amino acids you need. I'm talking about pork, fish, chicken, and turkey. These are fantastic sources, high in protein and low in fat.

2. **EGGS.** Those nine essential amino acids are also found in arguably the most popular breakfast food, eggs. There are countless ways to eat eggs, so get creative! They have so many great health benefits. Some of you may be worried about eating eggs since they are linked to cholesterol, and cholesterol is linked to heart health. Don't worry, I prefer egg whites. For the rest of you, know that the National Heart Foundation of Australia says eating up to six eggs per week will not increase your risk of heart disease.[1] By the way, eggs aren't just for breakfast. This idea that we can only have eggs in the morning has got to go, and I'm leading the charge. It's too good of a food for the body to eat just in the morning. You can

mix some egg whites with some veggies at night and have a delicious omelet . . . for DINNER. You'll get all those amino acids you need, plus you can add all the greens you want to your omelet.

3. **PROTEIN SUPPLEMENTS.** I'm cheating a bit here, but supplements can be a great way to get all the nine amino acids you need without any of the additives you don't. Whey, egg white, and pea protein are great additions to your diet, particularly when you're on the go. Protein powder is one of my favorite things to balance out my meal when I don't have the time or energy to cook an elaborate meal.

4. **SOYBEANS.** Although soybeans and quinoa are considered complete protein sources, I want you to think of them more as carbs than protein. Out of all the plants, soybeans are the only ones known as a complete protein, which is great, but there are some other things to consider, particularly if you're a man. Soy contains isoflavones, which act similarly to estrogen in the body. One study from the Harvard Medical School found that a nineteen-year-old on a vegan diet, high in soy, developed erectile dysfunction and hypogonadism (when the body doesn't produce enough testosterone).[2] Aside from the studies that link soy products with an increase in estrogen, they also contain lots of carbohydrates and fat. If you are trying to reach your protein levels with soybeans, you will have to eat such a large amount that you will be over your limit for carbs and fat. When I was vegetarian, I was eating lots of tofu and

tempeh to try to get my protein intake up, but I was gaining weight because of the carb and fat levels. Just keep in mind that although soybeans and quinoa are considered complete proteins, they fall more in line with our carb category.

5. QUINOA. Recent years have been kind to quinoa. I've noticed it popping up more and more on grocery store shelves and on the Food Network. With good reason, too. It has all nine of the amino acids the body needs, and it makes a great substitute for rice. It does have amounts of carbohydrates similar to brown rice, but it also contains more fiber and protein, so you will feel fuller for longer. Again, even though it's a complete protein source, I want you to think of it more as a carb than a protein. Got that? I'm only including it here because it's considered a complete protein with all nine of those amino acids, but you shouldn't fill your plate with quinoa trying to reach your protein numbers. It's not going to do you any favors on the scale.

Plenty of other foods are high in protein and contain essential amino acids, but those are the *complete sources* of protein. The incomplete proteins are things like peanut butter, beans, and dried peas. This brings me to one of the main criticisms people have of a vegetarian diet. The critics think that vegetarians need to combine protein sources for their meals, to essentially make a complete source of protein. However, I believe it is rarely a problem, as vegetarians typically eat a variety of foods that contain all of the nutrients the body needs.

We're all clear on the good proteins, yes? Good, because I want to explore what makes a bad protein. After all, we have good carbs and carbage, so shouldn't we talk about good protein versus bad? The main thing that separates good protein from bad protein, besides the ones that have all nine amino acids, is the saturated fat content. Foods high in saturated fat are known to eventually lead to heart disease, and we don't want that. Trust me, it's no fun. To avoid this, always go for the leaner meats. Red meat tends to be higher in saturated fat, which is why I recommend limiting red meat to two to three meals per month. When you do decide to eat a red meat, choose something lean. For instance, if you are cooking with ground beef, look for the package labeled "lean" or "extra lean." Oftentimes this will be marked as a percentage, and to be called "lean," it must be 92 percent lean or higher, meaning 8 percent fat or lower. If you are eating a red meat that is higher in fat, know that you won't be able to have the avocado with your meal because it will exceed your fat number.. Balance, as always, is key, and those numbers are going to keep you balanced. Want to know another great way to get lean protein with the right mix of amino acids? Protein powder! I previously mentioned that you can get a whole protein source from supplements, so I want to reiterate it here. There are countless varieties on the market, and sites like BulkApothecary .com sell egg white protein powder with zero preservatives or additives, which you can add to almond milk or water.

As always (I bet you already know what I'm going to say next), be mindful of the labels. Maybe I should've called this book *Be Mindful of the Labels*? The point is, you want to make sure you aren't buying something with a bunch of additives or preservatives, and there are tons of powders on the market with lots of junk added in. In fact, *Consumer Reports* tested protein powders back in 2010, and in fifteen powders and drinks they found several that had dangerous levels of arsenic, cadmium, or lead.[3] Read the labels before you buy to ensure that you aren't going to ingest something dangerous. Once you find a product you like, don't be afraid to turn a couple scoops of protein powder into a meal. If I'm running late for a meeting or a training session, it's nice to know I can throw some protein powder in my blender with almond milk or water, a dollop of peanut butter or handful of berries, shake it up, and walk out the door with something that is going to fill me up and get me going. Let's face it, some days we are going to have lots of time on our hands to make intricate and balanced meals, but other days we are going to need something fast and convenient.

I have the body I do—at fifty-one, no less—because of the mix of carbs, protein, and fat I put in it. If it wasn't for the *lean* protein

I eat, I wouldn't have the lean muscle mass that I have. I feel stronger and my muscles have the nutrients they need to grow and repair. My workouts are *tough*. I train using a mix of weights and cardio, and if I didn't have the right amount of protein, my body wouldn't be able to handle even half of what I do in the gym. This is true even when I was doing my cardiac rehab workouts. Think about the last time you had a tough training session with weights. If you pushed yourself, you probably had quite a bit of soreness in the targeted areas over the days that followed. Those aches and pains are the muscles breaking down. When you have the right protein, it will fill those muscles up so you can get back to the gym and continue training. It's like a deflated basketball. The protein is the air pump that is going to repair the deflated ball to get it ready to be used in the next game. Protein not only keeps your muscles pumped but it also gives you the essentials you need for strong hair, skin, and nails, it assists your immune system in fighting off bacteria, and it can even provide the energy your body needs when it isn't getting enough carbs. One of my goals in writing this book is to ensure that protein doesn't have to do that. Protein is already doing so much, I don't want it to have to be your main source of energy, too.

High-protein diets that have been all the rage in recent years rely on protein as a main source of energy. There are a lot of things I don't like about this type of diet, but one of the most alarming is the amount of fat that people take in while adhering to the plan. If you've considered these diets, or tried them yourself, you know that most of them recommend all the meat you can eat. They have no limits on how much fatty red meat you can eat, but they want you to give up carbs entirely. I've tried these diets and they never made much sense to me. It's simply too much fat with my protein. Now that I'm even more aware of my heart health, I'm seeing a different side to those other diet plans. It's not just about losing weight, remember? We want to be heart-healthy AND lose weight. That means limiting the amount of carbs, protein, AND fat. On the Super Carb Diet, I am making sure you aren't getting too much fat. Your fat grams are limited, just like your grams for protein and carbs. With the carbs back on your plate, you need to balance out your meals by taking away some of the fat that you are used to eating on some of the popular diets trending right now. The balance on your plate is going to get you to the weight you want, but it's not easy. These numbers are going to ensure that you are eating the good protein that is going to make you feel strong and healthy. And what about those other protein sources that are loaded with fat? They are going to hold you back in the gym, leave you feeling sluggish and overweight, and give your heart a hard time. I'm not banning red meat altogether, but I do want you to think twice before eating that steak. You really should only be having red meat once a month, a few times at most. And don't forget, if you do have a history of heart problems in your family, be sure to check with your doctor to see if you should be eating red meat at all. Your doctor needs this information to adjust your diet accordingly. I've included my own list of Super Carb Diet proteins below. These are the sources you should be looking for when you are grocery shopping and planning your meals.

SUPER PROTEINS

- Anchovies
- Beef (lean cuts)
- Bison
- Canadian bacon
- Casein powder
- Chicken breast
- Cottage cheese (nonfat)

- Eggs
- Egg white protein powder
- Greek yogurt (nonfat)
- Halibut
- Insects
- Lean ham
- Orange roughy
- Pea protein powder
- Pork
- Pork chops
- Pork loin
- Red snapper
- Sardines
- Sea bass
- Scallops
- Shrimp
- Steak (lean cuts; top or bottom round, filet)
- Swordfish
- Tilapia
- Tuna
- Turkey breast
- Turkey bacon
- Whey protein powder
- Yellowfin tuna

BAD PROTEINS

- Bacon
- Bologna
- Bratwurst
- Catfish
- Corned beef
- Fried chicken
- Hot dogs
- Lamb
- Salami
- Sausage

6.

ALL ABOUT FAT

You might assume I'm a millennial (don't roll your eyes), but I was, in fact, an adult in the 1980s. This means I lived through the whole fat-free craze that swept the nation. It all began when doctors started to warn the public that fat led to heart disease. Companies started slapping a "fat-free" label on everything. The problem is that taking out all of the fat required adding a lot of other ingredients. Most notably, sugar. I used to run around town with my bestie, eating a whole box of those cookies that were labeled fat-free. They were in a green box and had names like "Devil's Food Cake." Guess what? I wasn't getting any thinner. This brings me to our third macronutrient, fat.

We touched on fat in the last chapter because it's so closely related to those protein sources. Hopefully, by now you've learned that you must read beyond the buzzwords and look at the nutrition label. A bag of pretzels may be "fat-free," but that doesn't mean it's good for us or should be part of your Super Carb plate. What I mean is, fat grams are not the enemy. The body *requires* fat. Not only that, but fat is going to elevate your plate of food, making it look good and satisfying your taste buds. That doesn't mean I want you eating TOO much fat. I've been there, done that, when I did those no-carb diets. And guess what? Eating all that fat never made me feel strong. The idea of those other diets is that your body uses fat as a primary energy source instead of carbs, but as we talked about earlier, it isn't so simple. Instead, we're using what the body naturally wants to use as energy: carbs. We're still eating fat, but we're not eating such high amounts because we aren't using it as a fuel source. Let's look back at our Super Carb Diet fat numbers.

MEN: 15 grams of fat per meal

WOMEN: 12 grams of fat per meal

We know there's 9 calories in every gram of fat, which means, in caloric terms, 135 calories from fat per meal for men, and 108 calories from fat per meal for women. These numbers are obviously much lower than the ones for our protein and carbs, but that doesn't mean I want you to ignore them. I always think of the fat in my meal as my lifesaver. Without it, the food tends to be boring and unsubstantial. If I look at a salad without avocado, my brain dismisses it as not being enough food. If I add that avocado, I know I'm getting a substantial fat with my lettuce and it becomes much more visually appealing. I'm a visual person, so I need to see something tasty when I'm eating. However, it's not just about looks. Cooking with fat provides a nice texture for the food and prevents those lean meats from sticking to a pan or drying up. We've all tried to cook veggies or meat without any oil, only to ruin the food and order a pizza. Point is, a little fat goes a long way in making our meals look and taste appealing. There are some health benefits as well.

I know I said I didn't feel energized from fats when I was doing the no-carb thing, but I need to backtrack a bit. Fat is GREAT as energy storage. I don't want your body running solely off fat for its energy, but I am happy to see the healthy fats used properly. When you eat healthy fats, they will be stored in the fat tissue as energy. That stored fat will be used when your body needs it, like when you're doing one of my Body by Bob workouts.

Remember when we were talking about protein and I told you about the essential and nonessential amino acids? There's a similar situation with fat. The body needs fat for cell growth, to absorb nutrients, and to produce hormones. Without it, you would be malnourished. The body, being the great thing that it is, can produce almost all the necessary fatty acids on its own. There are two, however, it cannot produce: linoleic acid (LA) and alpha-linolenic acid (ALA). These are both vital to the body, and you can only get them from a proper diet. LA and ALA are also known as omega-6 and omega-3, respectively, and they are polyunsaturated fatty acids. You may even recognize linoleic acid from the ingredient label of your favorite beauty products. The point is, these fatty acids are important, and you need to get them from food.

Just as we broke down carbs and protein into different categories, we can do the same with fat. There are three different types of fats I want to focus on:

1. Unsaturated fat
    a. Monounsaturated
    b. Polyunsaturated
2. Saturated fat
3. Trans fat

The chemical structure of unsaturated fat is what distinguishes it from its saturated counterpart. Unsaturated has one or more double bonds (monounsaturated fats have one double bond, and polyunsaturated have more than one), while saturated fats have zero double bonds in their chemical structure. Most people, however, recognize unsaturated fats as the fat that is liquid at room temperature, while saturated is solid. The two types that the body doesn't make, LA and ALA, are polyunsaturated fats, meaning they have more than one double bond. Our third fat, trans fat, is made by a process called hydrogenation. Trans fat is typically artificial. Think margarine. It's fat that has been loaded with additives to make it last longer on the grocery store shelf. What I want you to know is that unsaturated fat is what we want and what the body needs. Saturated fat is what the body already makes, and trans fat is what I want you to avoid. Let's look at a nutrition label for one of my favorite fats, an avocado.

I want you to look at this graphic to help you understand the labels when you're shopping. And not just for the processed stuff. You can find nutritional information for all the

Nutrition Facts

Serving Size 1 avocado 201g (201 g)

Amount Per Serving

Calories 322	Calories from Fat 247

	% Daily Value*
Total Fat 29g	45%
Saturated Fat 4g	21%
Trans Fat	
Cholesterol 0mg	0%
Sodium 14mg	1%
Total Carbohydrate 17g	6%
Dietary Fiber 13g	54%
Sugars 1g	
Protein 4g	

Vitamin A	6%	•	Vitamin C	33%
Calcium	2%	•	Iron	6%

*Percent Daily Values are based on a 2,000 calorie diet. Your daily values may be higher or lower depending on your calorie needs.

foods, even one of my favorite fats, avocados. If you don't see it at the grocery, you can look it up online. You'll notice on the avocado label that the total fat is broken down to show how much saturated and trans fat is in it. Saturated and trans fats are both listed individually because they are required to be. Trans fats are so harmful that it is required *by law* to list them on a label individually. In this case, there's 4 grams of saturated fat and 0 grams of trans fat, so to get the total number of unsaturated fat, you would just subtract the 4 from the total fat grams (29). That gives us 25 grams of unsaturated fat in 1 avocado. Of course, on the Super Carb Diet, you're just looking at *total* grams, so if you were to eat the entire avocado, you would have eaten 29 grams of your fat total (way more than your allotted amount). You won't be able to eat an entire avocado with your meal at that fat content, but you can have some and save the rest for later. This is another example of how vital it is to READ THE NUTRITION LABELS on everything AND understand them.

SUPER TIP: When you're buying your extra-virgin olive oil or EVOO (Rachael Ray taught me well), make sure it is packaged in a dark bottle. This prevents the oil from going rancid.

The type of fat I want you to be eating most on the Super Carb Diet is the unsaturated. That means the foods with fewer grams of saturated and trans fat on the label. Now that you know how to differentiate the grams of fat, be sure to avoid the foods with a higher percentage of saturated or trans fat. We want the unsaturated ones.

One of the things I notice when people are trying to lose weight is that fat is the food they cut out first. Everyone thinks that when they are eating healthy, they need to cut out all the fat from their daily diet. This is setting yourself up for failure. If you don't have a healthy fat with your food, you will leave your dinner table unsatisfied. It's easy to throw some nuts on your salad or have a couple teaspoons of almond butter with your meal, so don't be afraid to do that. It's good for you! Remember, the body is SMART. When you don't eat enough fat the body gets confused. It will begin to store up fat just in case it needs it down the road because it knows you're not giving it enough. This is not going to be beneficial for you when you're trying to lose weight. You need fat, you just need to make sure it's the right amount and the right kind.

I've made a list of some of the fats I want you to avoid, alongside some of the fats I recommend on the Super Carb Diet. You may be looking at some of the oils in the bad fats and wondering why they fall under that category. The reason I want you to avoid them is they are misleading. These oils are often highly processed and infused with lots of chemicals, draining all the good stuff. What should you do to avoid them? ALWAYS CHECK THE NUTRITION LABEL. Read the ingredients, even on your oils, to make sure there are no added chemicals and you are getting the best product. Since we all like lists, I separated our good and bad fats into one comprehensive list for your grocery shopping pleasure. Enjoy!

BAD FATS

- Canola oil
- Corn oil
- Hydrogenated oils
- Margarine
- Safflower oil
- Soybean oil
- Vegetable oil

GOOD FATS

- Almonds
- Almond butter
- Avocado
- Chia seeds
- Coconut oil
- Edamame
- Egg yolks
  (in moderation)
- Extra-virgin olive oil
- Fish oils
- Flaxseed
- Flaxseed oil
- Ghee (get on the
  ghee train!)
- MCT oil
- Olive oil
- Olives
- Peanut butter
- Pistachios
- Pumpkin seed oil
- Pumpkin seeds
- Sardines/Mackerel (I
  wish I liked them!)
- Sunflower oil
- Sunflower seeds
- Walnuts

7.

LETTUCE TALK MORE
ABOUT VEGETABLES

Did you laugh at the chapter title? *Lettuce* Talk More About Vegetables . . . get it? It's cheesy, but we've done a lot of work to get here so I wanted to break the tension. I've thrown a LOT of information at you all up until this point. I don't want this process to be too painful. I mean, it's supposed to be hard, but it shouldn't be painstaking. You know what? Here's a picture of my dog, Karl. You've all earned it.

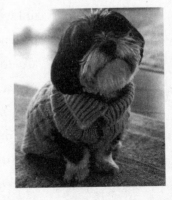

Isn't he adorable in that little doggie sweater? He is

just the sweetest and most chill dog in the world. Did I mention dogs are great for losing weight? It's basically forced exercise because you need to take them out for walks and play with them. They also provide companionship and unconditional love. I honestly don't know how I would've gotten through my heart attack recovery without Karl. Below is a picture of when we snuck him into my hospital room after my heart attack.

He brought me so much joy when I needed it most. He always does. If you're on the fence about getting a dog, just know your mental health will surely be improved if you adopt a rescue dog.

I hope that little diversion put you at ease with all this nutritional info I'm throwing your way. Even if it didn't, it's always fun to take a minute to look at dogs. As much as I would love to talk about Karl even more, we need to get back to this diet stuff. Specifically, I want to talk more about those vegetables we explored earlier. Why? Because on the Super Carb Diet you're allowed an extra 75 calories for your three main meals ON TOP OF all your carbs, protein, and fat. That means you can add a cup and a half of green beans, or a bell pepper, or a handful of baby carrots to the rest of your meal. I'm giving you so many vegetables for a reason: because they are great for you! It's hard to find fault with veggies, so I want you to fill your

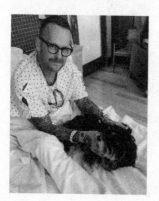

plate with as many as possible. Vegetables are loaded with vitamins and minerals that will boost your immune system, make your skin glow, satiate you, energize you, and more. Shall we dig deeper?

In the 2010 *Dietary Guidelines for Americans*, vegetables were broken down into five subgroups based on their nutrient content.[1]

1. Dark Green
2. Orange
3. Legumes
4. Starchy
5. Other Types

Vegetables are broken down this way because each category has different nutrients. For example, one would think that sweet potatoes and a regular potato would both be considered starch, but sweet potatoes are listed in the orange group, not just because of their coloring but because they contain substantially more vitamin A than a regular potato. The veggies are separated by their nutritional profile. That means not all green vegetables are listed in the dark green category and not all potatoes are considered equal, got it? The spectrum of veggies is also so vast that this helps us narrow them down further. On the Super Carb Diet, those 75 extra calories are going to come from my own cultivated list of the best veggies around. Before we get to that list, let's dig a little deeper.

The first category, dark green vegetables, are those leafy greens that you can eat and eat and eat on the Super Carb Diet without a care. This is the category I want you to load up on. The dark green vegetables are low in calories, high in fiber, and are great sources of vitamin A, C, and K, plus iron, folate, and calcium. If you're not sure what to make for a meal, use this category as your base and make a salad. These leafy greens are my absolute favorites. I want you to eat as many as possible and never feel like you must restrict the amount. There's not a whole lot better for you than a plate of dark greens, so eat up!

EXAMPLES OF DARK GREEN VEGETABLES

- Arugula
- Bok choy
- Broccoli
- Collard greens
- Kale
- Lettuce
- Mustard greens
- Spinach
- Turnip greens
- Watercress

The second category is your orange vegetables. This includes—you guessed it—the orange ones. You may have heard people say that carrots are good for the eyes, and they're right. Carrots and other orange vegetables are rich in vitamin A, vitamin C, and lutein, which are imperative for good eye health. They also promote collagen formation, fight harmful free radicals in your body, boost your immune system, and lower blood pressure. Red peppers taste great when they're dipped in hummus. (Just remember to count the carbs in that hummus toward your totals.) The orange vegetables are fantastic and the flavor profiles are incredibly robust. You can crisp sweet potatoes in an air fryer for fries, mash some pumpkin and make some protein bars, or roast some carrots and squash for a delicious side dish.

EXAMPLES OF ORANGE VEGETABLES

- Carrots
- Pimiento
- Pumpkin
- Tomato (I know tomatoes are *technically* a fruit, but you'll find them by the veggies in the grocery store and we're using them as a veggie on the Super Carb Diet.)
- Red pepper
- Squash
- Sweet potato

The legume (god I hate that word) category is beans and peas. These are loaded with dietary fiber, which you know I love, plus legumes are cholesterol-free. You'll find lots of folate and potassium; however, 75 calories are not going to go a long way with legumes.

EXAMPLES OF LEGUMES

- Black beans
- Chickpeas
- Kidney beans
- Lentils
- Navy beans
- Pinto beans
- Red beans
- Soy beans
- Split peas
- White beans

Starchy vegetables are next, and they are also rich in fiber and complex carbohydrates. You may be wondering why green lima beans are considered a starch and not found in the legume category. That's because green lima beans have more complex carbohydrates, making them fall under the starch subgroup with like-minded veggies. These vegetables are great sources of B vitamins, which, according to the Harvard School of Public Health, may help lower your risk for heart disease and stroke.[2] They are also very high in calories and carbs, so limit your intake and watch your numbers with them.

P.S. If you're a chip eater and want a healthy alternative to starchy and fried potato chips, I recommend kale chips. They're sold at most major grocery chains, and they give you that salty crunch. Just make sure you're buying a brand without lots of additives. You may be thinking, "But Bob, how will I do that?" READ THE LABELS (or make your own at home).

EXAMPLES OF STARCHY VEGETABLES

- Black-eyed peas
- Cassava
- Corn
- Green bananas
- Green lima beans
- Green peas

- Jicama
- Plantains
- Potatoes
- Taro
- Water chestnuts

Finally, our "other" category is filled with the beautiful rainbow of vegetables that march to the beat of their own drum. Some of these are starchy or green, but the USDA categorizes them in the "other" category because they don't have the same nutrition profiles as the others. Remember, it's not just the color of a vegetable that tells you where it falls. These vegetables don't match the nutrients of the others, but that doesn't mean they are bad. Far from it. They are heart-healthy foods that contain lots of vitamin C and help improve immunity. I'm a fan of most of the veggies in this category. Just remember, we do have a calorie restriction with our extra veggies, so be aware. Be mindful of the serving size and use your food scale.

EXAMPLES OF OTHER VEGETABLES

- Artichokes
- Asparagus
- Bean sprouts
- Beets
- Brussels sprouts
- Cabbage
- Cauliflower

- Celery
- Eggplant
- Garlic
- Green peppers
- Okra
- Mushrooms
- Onion

- Radishes
- Turnips
- Wax beans

- Yellow summer squash
- Zucchini

I list a lot of vegetables, both in this chapter and in previous ones. I did that so you can see their names, right in front of you, and hopefully start to explore some options you haven't tried before. People get in ruts. Usually I talk about ruts when it comes to working out, but it happens with food, too. We tend to eat the same stuff. You get in the habit of going to the grocery store, picking up some broccoli, coming home, steaming it, and repeating a few days later. To be honest, that works for me, but it may not work for you. I am a creature of habit. I like having the same meals often. It keeps me disciplined, but I understand it's not for everyone. And I don't want you to get in a rut or give up, thinking you don't have options. Look at the lists of vegetables I've laid out for you. Find a vegetable you haven't tried before and seek it out at the store. You may like it, you may not, but experimenting will get you out of your rut or keep you out of one. It will ensure that your taste buds are constantly engaged and keep you from going stir crazy.

I can't come into your kitchen and cook with you. I wish I could. I can, however, remind you that you need to make sure you're spicing things up on the Super Carb Diet. Don't become complacent, because it will set you up for failure. You have all the rules for eating on the Super Carb Diet in front of you (we'll get to the other guidelines next), so now it's up to you to get to work at the grocery store and in your kitchen.

On the Super Carb Diet, I want you to craft your plate focusing on carbs, protein, fat, and vegetables and using the numbers you calculated for your specific body. You should *always* have a vegetable on your plate. But, and this is a big but, it's possible to put together a meal without any vegetables at all. If you do, it's not going to be a whole lot of food. That's why I'm giving you 75 extra calories from vegetables. I am doing absolutely everything I can to ensure that you start adding more vegetables to your diet. It is going to completely change your relationship with food. The more veggies you eat, the healthier you'll be. I see it all the time. When clients start eating more vegetables, the junk that they used to eat, slowly but surely, starts to fall by the wayside. Why? Because they aren't hungry. Filling up on greens and squash is going to keep you fuller, longer, and stop you from filling up on all the crap. Are there some vegetables I would rather have you eat than others? Yes. In a perfect world, you wouldn't be eating a regular potato with every meal, but the numbers are going to keep you in check in terms of your protein, carbs, and fat. You'll find that the good naturally overcomes the bad when it comes to vegetables. For the extra 75 calories, I want you to select from the list I created of Super Carb Veggies. It's the same list I laid out earlier when I talked about carbs. It's the best of the best. If you stay within those carb, protein, and fat numbers we calculated earlier, plus the extra 75 calories from the veggies I have listed, you will not gain weight. One last thing: please remember you don't HAVE to eat the extra 75 calories. It's okay if you don't. These numbers are your caps. If you made a whole meal filled with veggies that fit into your Super Carb equation for carbs, protein, and fat WITHOUT the extra 75 calories of veggies, don't worry about stuffing your face with them just because I said you can. If you do, stick to the ones in this list and you'll be golden.

SUPER CARB VEGGIES

- Artichokes
- Arugula
- Asparagus
- Beets
- Bell peppers
- Bok choy
- Broccoli
- Broccoflower
- Broccoli romanesco
- Brussels sprouts
- Butternut squash
- Cabbage
- Carrots
- Cauliflower
- Chard
- Chinese cabbage
- Collard greens
- Cucumbers
- Curly endive
- Daikon
- Dandelion
- Eggplant
- Escarole
- Ethiopian mustard
- Fennel
- Garlic
- Green beans
- Horseradish
- Iceberg lettuce
- Jicama
- Kale
- Kohlrabi
- Komatsuna (Japanese mustard spinach)
- Leeks
- Lettuce
- Mâche
- Mizuna
- Mushrooms
- Mustard greens
- Onions
- Parsnips
- Pumpkin
- Radishes
- Rutabaga
- Scallions
- Spinach
- Tatsoi
- Tomatoes
- Turnips
- Watercress
- Wild broccoli
- Yams
- Yellow summer squash
- Zucchini

8.

WHAT TO DO WHEN YOU WANT TO CHEAT

D^{on't.}

9.

TIPS AND TRICKS

Are we clear on the fact that I don't want you to cheat on this diet? It's only ninety days. I know that may seem like a while right now, but in the grand scheme of things it's nothing. Years go by in the blink of an eye. Hell, it seems like only yesterday I was teaching a hip-hop cardio class as a twentysomething who had just moved to LA. You all would have loved my class! I made sure everyone was sweating and laughing. I digress. The point is, I don't want you cheating. People are always looking for the easy way out, and there is none. Sometimes you need to put in the work. This is one of those times. There are going to be some situations you find yourself in where you are tempted to cheat. I'm going to go through as many of those as I can with some tips and tricks on how to avoid the temptation.

VACATIONS

This is a big one. It's hard to eat healthy on a vacation. I want you cooking your own meals, which is going to be tough if you're on vacation. Not only that, but if you're traveling to a place you've never been, you're going to want to try the local foods. And you should! If you have a trip planned to Italy or India, save the Super Carb Diet for when you get back. Don't miss out on trying once-in-a-lifetime meals just for me. If you decide to hold off on going all-in on the Super Carb Diet, there are a few things you can do to make sure you don't gain tons of weight on your time away from home.

1. **DON'T OVEREAT.** When you're out to dinner, eat slowly. Usually when people overeat, it's because they are inhaling their food. Eating slowly will help you determine if and when you are full. I don't want to deprive you of food when you're on vacation, but I also don't want you to eat everything in sight. Be selective.

2. **DIP YOUR TOE IN BEFORE JUMPING IN THE WATER.** This is a metaphor for eating. When you're on vacation, you're going to be presented with all sorts of new foods you may not have back home. You should try new things, but don't order a full plate of everything. If you're with friends or family, try a bite off everyone's plate instead of ordering your own serving of each thing. This will stop you from eating things you don't like just because they are in front of you. We've all been there,

right? There's something you aren't even enjoying, but you eat a whole plate just because you feel bad letting it go to waste.

3. **FIND FITNESS.** Whether you're on a beach in the Bahamas or near a slot machine in Vegas, there is always time to get in a workout. I like to carry a jump rope with me because I know I can get a great cardio burn in with little space if I just have a hotel gym or a beach at my disposal. If you don't want to dedicate time for a traditional workout, find an activity that will keep you moving. Swimming, hiking, and shopping can be great ways to get some steps in while you're away from home. You've heard it before, and I'm going to tell you again: take the stairs! At the very least, while you're away, take the stairs when it's an option. If you don't do anything else that's active on your vacation, please just take the stairs wherever you can. P.S. I included a hotel workout at the end of this book, so there's no excuse!

HOLIDAYS

Holidays are tough on our bodies. People celebrate with food, so anytime a holiday comes up, we are faced with tons of temptation. Thanksgiving to New Year's has become a month-and-a-half-long celebration of stuffing pumpkin and peppermint everything in our mouths. This past year, spring has become the unofficial unicorn time of year where colorful "unicorn" foods with loads of artificial ingredients are popping up everywhere. Of course, summer is rosé season. Then there's Valentine's Day dinners, Halloween candy, and Super Bowl Sunday appetizers. Chances are there will be some holiday that falls within the ninety days you are doing the Super Carb Diet. If you're hosting a holiday party, center it on an activity rather than the dinner table. Cover the dinner table with Monopoly or a hot glue gun and glitter if you have to, just don't use it for eating all the time.

1. **DON'T CELEBRATE WITH FOOD.** If you're hosting a holiday party, center it on an activity rather than the dinner table. I know we're all used to setting up parties around food, but there are other options. Make some healthy snacks that fit into your Super Carb plate, and then have something for the guests to do BESIDES eat. Cooking is a hobby, but eating is not.

2. **SHOW UP LATE.** This is something many of you probably do already. I'm a very punctual person. I hate being late, and you should, too. I'm not advocating that you be one of those people who walks into a function whenever they please. Instead, I'm telling you to inform the host or the other guests that you will be arriving late so you will be missing the meal. If you know there is a cocktail hour before the food is served, I recommend arriving early and planning an exit before the dinner starts. Either way, you can have a good time mingling with friends and family, but you won't be eating a bunch of garbage food that is going to throw you off track.

3. **BYOSCF.** This stands for "Bring Your Own Super Carb Food." Chances are you will be bringing something to that party you're headed to anyway. If you aren't, you should. Even if the host tells you not to, it's still the polite thing to do. If you're planning on bringing a side dish

or appetizer, make something that you can eat alongside something you make for everyone else. It may feel a little bit like you're packing a lunch for a social gathering, but it will be much easier to resist the foods everyone else is eating if you have your own food that is Super Carb–approved. You can even make a Super Carb dish that you like for everyone else. I find that most people like healthy food when they're presented with it, so share the love and get other people on board with your new eating habits.

4. **DON'T SHOP HUNGRY.** Holiday gift shopping can be an all-day event. Eat before you leave, or have your meal already prepared for you when you get home. If you're spending the day at the mall or driving from store to store, you're likely to lose all inhibitions and pick up some unhealthy snacks along the way. That's when people make bad decisions like drive-thrus and pretzel-wrapped hot dogs. Never shop hungry. This tip is also applicable to grocery shopping. Always grocery shop after a meal so you make smart decisions. Don't let hunger lead you astray.

STRESS

Who hasn't stress-eaten a bag of potato chips in their lifetime? We've all had a bad breakup, sudden death in the family, or a boss that won't cut you a break. Next thing you know, you're crying in the bathtub with Adele on repeat, a bag of tortilla chips by your side, and a bottle of merlot against your lips. Tale as old as time. There are some ways to fight this instinct.

1. **BREATHE.** I'm a big proponent of meditation. Taking the time to connect your brain with your body every day is incredibly beneficial to your overall mental health. However, even if you aren't versed in meditation, you can always take a few seconds to breathe. Usually when a craving hits, we begin to think about satisfying that craving. Your thoughts race as you think about the smell of the food you are craving, or the texture. Your mind is consumed with giving in to that craving. In those moments when you are impulsively reaching for the junk food, stop and close your eyes. Ask yourself if it's worth it and if there is a better choice you can make. Breathe. Taking a few moments will slow those thoughts about cravings down to a manageable pace.

2. **REDIRECT.** Stress eating is a slippery slope. Once you have that one candy bar, you're going to be more likely to eat garbage food the rest of the day. In those moments of weakness, redirect your impulse to another vice. That doesn't mean I want you to grab a cigarette. But you can buy yourself something nice, like some new clothes, or even treat yourself to a spa day. Find something that will calm you down without involving food.

3. **EXERCISE.** There's no better stress reliever than exercise! Next time you are feeling frantic, head to the nearest gym. Even if you've already worked out, there's no harm in hopping on the treadmill at a slow pace to calm your nerves. The endorphin rush will help level you out and keep you out of the kitchen. Even if it's a quick walk outside (vitamin D!) or a slow bike ride, exercising will clear your head so that you can take your mind off

food and think about things with a fresh perspective. Personally, I like yoga to deal with my stress. It incorporates all these ideas—breathing, exercise, and redirection. It's been essential to my mental recovery from the heart attack. I look at yoga with fresh eyes. Now, I use it as a time to clear my mind of all the negative chatter.

One of the things I realized when I was healing from my heart attack is that I can be a very sarcastic person. Some of that is my sense of humor, but some of it was a defense mechanism. I was recently talking to my bestie, Cristi, about a certain television personality joining a talk show. I was making jokes at that person's expense. It wasn't a good look on me. Normally I would've gotten off the phone and not thought anything of it. Instead, I recognized that my comments were coming from a place of jealousy. I called Cristi back. She's a friend that loves me no matter what, so I wasn't calling for her. I was calling for me. I needed to hold myself accountable and call myself out on that behavior. It's become important to me to make sure my actions match my intentions.

I would have never recognized that behavior if it weren't for yoga. I've learned to see that side of myself in a different light. Connecting the physical to the mental has allowed me to see things I have never seen before. Not only that, but surviving something life-threatening gives you a whole new perspective of the world. Now I embrace each moment, so when I'm practicing yoga I can enjoy wherever I am instead of thinking about where I should be. I say this all to let you know that exercise is crucial to stress management. It's great to look at a gym and think about how it is going to help shape your body into the physical shape that you are striving for. However, I challenge you all to start looking at a gym (or a yoga studio), and thinking about how it can shape you mentally. It does both, but it's up to you to refocus your thinking.

INJURIES

When you're injured, it's easy to get discouraged and quit. You think, "I can't go to the gym anyway, so what's the point of trying to diet?" When you hurt yourself, it's even MORE important to make sure your eating habits are solid. After my heart attack, I was forced to put my gym membership on hold. Doctor's orders. I was fortunate enough to have experts monitoring my diet, so even though I wasn't working out like my body was used to, I was still able to maintain my weight. Too often I see people have a physical setback that creates a domino effect. The weight piles on quickly, and once it does, people lose ALL inhibitions. Suddenly, you're a hundred pounds (or more) overweight, all because of an injury. Guess what? Losing inhibitions is not going to help you heal quicker. Quite the opposite. If you maintain a healthy and balanced diet, your body will have the resources it needs to heal. You'll heal quicker *and* prevent weight gain. Here's how to survive a new injury when you're on the Super Carb Diet:

1. **FIND ALTERNATIVE EXERCISE.** You won't believe how many times I've had clients tell me they can't exercise because of a foot injury, or an elbow issue. You can (almost) ALWAYS exercise. You just need to get creative. That means finding a stationary bike if your arms are hurt, or carefully chest pressing with a broken foot. The pool is a great way to work out if you're rehabbing a part of your body that was recently injured. Not sure

what to do? Ask one of the trainers or staff at your gym. There are so many options and there's always people around to guide you. Don't be shy!

2. **EAT LESS**. If you're not working out, or working out with less intensity than normal, you don't need as much food as you normally do. Remember, food is fuel. If you are spending the day in bed because of an accident, then you shouldn't be eating the same number of carbs, protein, and fat you do on an average day. The problem is that people get used to eating a certain amount of food. This happens on the Super Carb Diet just like it does for people who aren't on the plan. You must adjust your portions if you are inactive. Look, I know that injuries happen that are out of your control. You may not be able to make it to the gym at all, or your doctor may advise you against it. In these instances, you must be diligent about your food intake and make sure you don't over-eat. Those numbers we mapped out are a cap. Adjust down if you are unable to exercise.

Your goal on the Super Carb Diet should be ninety days of uninterrupted meal planning and exercise. That's how you will get the very best results. However, I understand that life happens. It is my goal to give you all the tools you need to be successful. On *TBL*, there are teams of people with the contestants every step of the way. I can't be with you all 24/7, but I'm giving you all the information you need to do it on your own. But I need you to be diligent and tough. A lot of that is going to come down to will-power. How much do you have? In those moments when you want to cheat, you must have the willpower to say no and keep moving forward. It's going to be hard! We all have moments of weakness. Resist. I'm fifty-one years old. Believe me, it doesn't get easier as you get older. If anything, it gets tougher. If you get off track for a couple of weeks in your teens or twenties, it's easy to drop the weight quickly. As you get older, it gets harder and harder. Those times when you cheat are more difficult to make up for the older you get, so don't form those habits now. We talk a lot about habits when we talk about diet and exercise because we know that consistency is key for success. Forming habits now will help you later. That's true in diet, exercise, and even sleep. Which leads me to my next rule: sleep. After all, the Super Carb Diet isn't just about food and exercise.

10.

SLEEPING YOUR WAY TO HEALTHY

Until now, I've been focusing on all the things you need to eat or not eat on the Super Carb Diet. The plate is the most important thing, but it's not *every*thing. You may have heard me on TV talking about the pillars of health. These pillars are what you need to have stability in your life: diet, sleep, exercise, and stress management. That second one is vital. We need sleep. It's going to give you the strength you need to get through this plan alive! On the Super Carb Diet, I want you to get seven to nine hours of sleep. Every night. Every. Single. Night. This is super important and will be the key to achieving your goals. Do not ignore this pillar. I know there's been lots of rules thus far, and you're tired. It's a lot to take in,

I know. But sleep is beneficial to your success. If you're reading this in bed, I want you to put this book down and go to sleep right now so you can get seven to nine hours. Go ahead. I'll wait.

Now, I'm assuming you got seven to nine hours and you're ready to continue the Super Carb journey you started. If not, I need you to put an effort into adhering to this rule. Why? Because no one is sleeping enough. I know many reasonably healthy people that don't get enough sleep and run into all sorts of problems. There's a reason for their troubles. Sleep is fundamental and your body needs the rest to heal. I want you working out on this plan, and that means your body will be fatigued. Even if you never set foot in a gym, your body still needs the sleep. And it's not just about sleeping so you're rested for the gym every day. In 2010, the journal *Sleep* published a study of over a thousand twins. Researchers found that the twin who slept less than seven hours per night had a higher body mass index than the twin who slept more than nine hours.[1] I'm not advocating for all of you to sleep more than nine hours, but it's important that you don't sleep less than seven. A proper night's sleep of seven to nine hours is going to help you lose weight.

Have you ever had one of those nights when you barely slept and then spent the next day eating everything in sight? I have, and there's a couple different reasons this happens.

1. **MENTAL ALERTNESS.** This is the most obvious reason. When you lack sleep, your brain is groggy. I don't know about you, but when I'm groggy, I don't have the patience to be adding up numbers or to keep track of my macronutrients. I'm much more likely to have the bag of tortilla chips for breakfast instead of the egg whites with peppers. Think about when you have a hangover.

Usually when you've been drinking, your sleep sucks. You don't get enough and it's not quality. You wake up the next day and all you want to do is stuff your face with food. You don't care what you ingest because your brain is foggy and your body/mind is telling you it wants junk. Keep your brain sharp and you'll make better decisions.

2. **HORMONES.** If you're tired, your body will produce extra ghrelin, which is the hormone that tells you when you're hungry, and a tired body will also produce less leptin, the hormone that tells you when you're full. Combined, the imbalance will cause you to be hungry and unsatisfied. We don't want that. That's how you end up reaching for the chocolate chip cookies. In fact, the *American Journal of Clinical Nutrition* published a study which found that sleep-deprived patients eat, on average, 300 calories more per day.[2] You can't argue with science.

A proper night's rest will give you the strength you need at the gym and in the kitchen. So, you're reading this and thinking, "This all sounds great, Bob, but how am I going to get more sleep? I'm busy!" I'm busy, too. However, I prioritize. I know how important sleeping is to my overall health. Here's what I do:

1. **KEEP WORK OUT OF YOUR BEDROOM.** Thanks to the internet and mobile phones, we can all work 24/7. We can answer emails while we watch the housewives of Beverly Hills, New York, Atlanta, Dallas, Orange County, Potomac, and more. We can have FaceTime conference calls in our pajamas, all the while cozied up in our beds. While convenient, it's not ideal. Your bedroom should

be a sacred sleeping space. If you bring work into your bed, then your body and mind will start to think of it like an office. The body and mind are smart, and if you keep acting like your bed is a conference table, you will start to believe it. I try my best to keep all my activity outside my bedroom, even watching TV. I know that's hard to do when it's so easy to pull up old seasons of *The Biggest Loser* on your iPad and see how my hair has changed through the years. I try my best to keep the dramas and reality shows in the living room. That way, when it's time to go to bed my body and mind know that as soon as I hit my pillow, I'm ready to get some shut-eye. There is one activity in the bedroom when it's okay to break the rules, and it is a *wonderful* calorie burn. I highly recommend doing it as much and as safely as possible. I'll let you use your imagination.

2. **THAT MEANS SOCIAL MEDIA, TOO.** Turn off Twitter at a set time every night. Give your brain a break. Look, I love social media and being able to interact with all you guys, but we need to have limits. Social media is now a twenty-four-hour thing, and it's too easy to grab your phone in bed and check your timeline. You do it, I do it, and even the people that say they don't do it . . . they do it, too. But you (we) need to stop. So, stop! . . . Unless you want to tweet me (@MyTrainerBob) something nice about the book (#SuperCarbDiet). That's an exception. Or if you want to like one of my Instagram (@BobHarper) photos. Or follow me on Facebook (@MyTrainerBob). Or follow my friend and co-writer, Danny, on Instagram and Twitter (@DannyPellegrino).

He's hilarious. Did you get all that? Me or Danny is all that's allowed. And only nice things. Other than that, SHUT IT DOWN!

3. **BEDTIME.** You thought bedtime was done once you reached puberty, but it shouldn't be. It's the same reasoning as making your bedroom strictly a sleeping room. You must train your body and your mind. It's one of those habits you should be forming. If you adhere to a set schedule, then you will find it easier to go to sleep every night. This is particularly important on the Super Carb Diet, when sleep loss is so detrimental. Follow a schedule as closely as possible. By the way, for the parents out there, this is also important for your children. Getting them on a set sleeping schedule is just as important for them as it is for yourself. Your kids also need the same tools to be successful in their eating.

4. **CUT THE CAFFEINE.** I love an espresso after dinner, but I know that if I have one too late at night, I will have trouble closing my eyes. Some of you may not be caffeine-sensitive, but if you are, you need to stop drinking caffeine in the late afternoon or early evening. Opt for decaf or an herbal tea.

5. **INVEST IN YOUR BED.** Hello! You spend half your life in your bedroom, you should invest in it. I know people like to spend their money in the living room, which everyone can see, but the bedroom is, in my opinion, even more important. Buy some fancy sheets, purchase a new mattress, and get some plush pillows. There is nothing better than a good mattress. Do whatever it takes to make the room as inviting as possible. If you

want to be in the room, you'll want to get in bed. Plus, if you want to be in the bedroom, chances are other people will want to be in the bedroom as well, so you'll have the chance for some of that extra calorie-burning cardio I alluded to earlier.

6. **EXERCISE.** If your body is worn out, you'll want to sleep. I promise. Do one of the Body by Bob workouts in this book, and you'll want nothing more than to crawl into bed.

A good night's rest will carry you through those times of weakness when you want to give up. Most diets I've done have a list of things you should and shouldn't eat, but they often forget to mention sleep. It's crucial that you get enough on the Super Carb Diet. I know you're busy. You have jobs, and kids, and now you need to worry about cooking and working out. It's a lot. But without sleep, everything else will crumble. You won't have the energy to follow the rest of the rules or the motivation to keep going. If you are the type of person that is normally getting six to seven hours of sleep, I want you to negotiate some of your other areas of life so you are getting a solid seven hours. That doesn't mean six hours and fifty minutes. It's seven to nine hours. Every night. Start thinking of this as a part of your diet for the next ninety days. It's a Super Carb rule from here on out. Got it? Now get some rest and come back after you do. We still have more to talk about!

11.

THE FOURTH MACRO

You know everything there is to know about macro-nutrients, right? We covered carbs, protein, and fat. What else is there? Almost everything we eat or drink falls into one of those three categories. Not so fast. There is something we haven't talked about that doesn't quite fit alongside our main three of carbs, protein, and fat. I'm talking about booze. That's why, in some circles, you may hear alcohol referred to as the fourth macronutrient. Believe me, on some nights, alcohol is the most important macronutrient.

Do I recommend drinking on the Super Carb Diet? No. Alcohol is high in calories and leads to bingeing on food. Drinking is not good on a diet. Have you ever been drunk and near New York City pizza? It's almost impossible to order just one slice when you're walking home from a night out with friends. Plus, a hangover is going to lead to lots of bad food decisions on day two. Furthermore, when you're counting your macronutrients for each meal, there's no easy way to calculate alcohol. So, don't drink for ninety days.

That said, I'm going to show you a way to drink on the Super Carb Diet, but it's convoluted and insanely mathematical. If you thought the basic Super Carb math was hard, you aren't going to like this. If you do drink, I need you to know how to factor it into your daily diet so you don't get too far off track and can keep losing weight. Where there's a will, there's a way. This chapter is all about the special occasion that may lead you astray. You can calculate alcohol into your Super Carb plate when you absolutely, one-hundred-percent MUST have a cocktail. Hopefully, you'll use this calculation sparingly during your ninety days. If you've completed the diet, but want to continue to eat and drink as intelligently as you can, then you can grab this book off the shelf and open this chapter before a night out and get some tips and tricks when it comes to drinking. Let's recap a few macronutrient facts that are going to be relevant to alcohol.

Remember this?

1 gram of carbohydrates = 4 calories

1 gram of protein = 4 calories

1 gram of fat = 9 calories

That's our gram-to-calorie equation for carbs, protein, and fat. If you're looking at a nutrition label and the food at hand has 2 grams of carbohydrates, we know that it has 8 calories because 1 gram of carbohydrates is 4 calories ($4 \times 2 = 8$). You probably thought you were done with math, and here I come in chapter 11 like your fourth-grade math teacher haunting your dreams. Losing weight is hard and I will not apologize for it!

That fourth "macronutrient," alcohol, technically looks like this:

1 gram of alcohol = 7 calories

If you look back on your caloric numbers for every meal, you'll see they were broken down into calories of carbs, protein, and fat. But alcohol isn't a carb, a protein, or a fat. It's not a nutrient at all (which is why I don't want you having any if you can help it). So how many alcohol calories or grams are you allotted per meal or per day? Technically, none. Particularly when you are starting this program. But if you're going to do it, I'd prefer it to be under my supervision. I sound like a parent, don't I? Maybe that's why so many people call me Daddy on Instagram? Regardless, I'm done with the alcohol disclaimers. Proceed at your own risk.

Since you don't NEED alcohol with your meal, we need to subtract the alcohol calories from your allotted *carbs* per meal. Why from the carbs and not the protein or fat? Most importantly, because it's easiest. It's a bit more scientifically accurate to count it toward your carbohydrates AND fats, but that gets tricky and we're already doing enough math. Besides, carbohydrates are the most flexible of all your numbers. Your body *needs* the protein and fat even more than carbohydrates, so the wiggle room happens in the carb category. If you are having an alcoholic beverage, I want you to calculate the calories and subtract them from the calories per meal you are eating for carbs. Calculating alcohol macros is certainly not ideal or exact, but we can get close. Does this make sense? Let's remind you of my numbers per meal:

1. 160 calories from carbs per meal.
2. 136 calories from protein per meal.
3. 135 calories from fat per meal.

If I have alcohol, I'll be factoring the alcohol calories from the 160 calories (or 40 grams) I'm having for carbs per meal. Got it? Here's that same list as grams per meal:

1. 40 grams of carbs per meal.
2. 34 grams of protein per meal.
3. 15 grams of fat per meal.

When consuming alcohol, I want you to subtract the grams from your *daily* total of carbs. That means alcohol, for me, would only be factored in with the 160 calories (aka 40 grams) from carbs per meal. Even though the drinking will be most likely happening at night (right?), I want you to subtract from your total grams of carbs for the entire *day*. This takes a little extra math and planning, but it's ideal for you to have a game plan for the drinking occasion. If you know you're going out with friends and you want to have one or two drinks, you can use this information to plan your day ahead of time.

Circling back, we see that I'm eating about 160 total grams of carbs per day (40 grams for each meal, 3 times a day). If I have a glass of alcohol that is 100 calories, I divide that by 4 (because there are 4 calories in every gram of carbohydrates), and I get 25. That means I would be factoring 25 grams of carbs from that one drink from my DAILY total. Having that one drink means I should be having 95 grams of carbs total for the day ASIDE FROM that glass of alcohol. Did you see how I got this?

Total number of grams of carbs per meal = 40 grams

Total number of grams of carbs per day = 120 grams

100-calorie drink = 25 grams of carbs

120 − 25 = 95 grams of carbs left over

Finally, we divide the 95 by 3 (because there's 3 meals per day where I'm factoring in carbs), which leaves us 31 (rounded down) grams of carbs per meal on the day we are having that one alcoholic beverage. Is it worth it? Just having one drink per day will cut my carbs per meal down from 40 grams to 31 grams. And that's only one drink!! That's a substantial amount. It's up to you to decide if it's worth it. Some days, it might be.

You can also calculate using your caloric totals, and it becomes (a little) easier. If you are having a 100-calorie glass of wine, simply subtract that 100 calories from the 480 calories of carbs per day (160 calories from carbs per meal, 3 meals with carbs per day). You'll see that this leaves you with very little left over. Just one glass of wine is going to substantially reduce the number of carbs you're allotted for that day. You need to plan, do extra math, AND restrict your eating. With such a limited number of calories from carbs left over, you'll have to forgo that slice of bread at dinner or that rice. Plus, eating less at dinner means you'll get drunk quicker, so your hangover is going to be worse. You'll also run the risk of binge eating when your inhibitions are lowered. You see why I don't want you drinking on the Super Carb Diet? It can throw everything off balance, and WE NEED BALANCE.

SUPER CARB DRINKS

1. **TEQUILA.** Tequila is sugar-free, low-carb, and comes from a plant. If you buy the right kind. That means what? You guessed it, read the labels! A 1 ounce shot is around 65 calories, depending on the type and brand. If you have a choice, always drink a tequila that is 100 percent agave. Otherwise, you will be consuming something with added sugars that aren't so good. P.S. Be careful not to let one shot of tequila lead to a margarita in round two . . . it's a slippery slope.

2. **POTATO VODKA.** This type of vodka, obviously, comes from potatoes, which is good. Like tequila, it's going to be sugar-free and low-carb if you buy the right kind. Just watch your mixers. Juice is going to put your carbs over your daily limit faster than you can count your macronutrients. For the tequila and potato vodka remember that mixers come with calories!

3. **RED WINE.** No mixers needed. Great for the heart. Simple. Classic. Be sure to get something dry since those varietals will contain minimal amounts of sugar.

I want you to stay away from absolutely everything else. Drinks like beer are very high in calories *and* carbs. You might think opting for a light beer would be okay, but those light beers are so stripped of flavor that people end up drinking more to get the effects they desire. That's another reason why I like red wine over beer (or white wine): because the flavor is so robust that you can enjoy one glass without craving much more. Don't do it unless it's worth it.

THE NO'S

- Beer
- White wine
- Liqueurs
- Margaritas
- Mojitos

- Mudslides
- Piña coladas
- Wine coolers
- Mixers!!

12.

MICRONUTRIENTS

The Super Carb Diet revolves around three macronutrients: carbs, protein, and fat. Macros are important, but we don't want to forget about micros. Micronutrients are necessary for the body, but only in very tiny amounts. In the protein section, we discussed protein supplements. Whey, pea, and egg white protein powders are fantastic options for getting the right amount and type of protein to help you build strong, lean muscles. The aisle at the grocery store where you'll find those wonderful powders is where you'll also find the micronutrients you need for optimum health.

People always ask me what supplements I take. There's so much information being thrown at us about which vitamins to take, it's overwhelming. Just like "carb," "supplement" has become a dirty word. People associate supplements with harmful chemicals and steroid use, but that's not how they should be thought of or used. We need supplements because, even though we are eating a balanced diet of healthy foods, we simply cannot get all the nutrients we need from our grub. Nowadays food has been pumped and stripped of vitamins and minerals. The way food is created is not what it used to be. Therefore, certain micronutrients we simply will not get unless we get them in pill or powder form. That doesn't mean we need to swallow a million pills every day, but there are some I recommend over others. The only real way to know which supplements you should be taking is to get your blood work done and find out what you may be deficient in. Here are the ones I take.

1. **MULTIVITAMIN.** A great daily multivitamin is crucial. If you only take one vitamin or supplement from this list, make sure it's the multivitamin. There are countless options when you go shopping for a multivitamin, but the main thing you want to look for is 100 percent of vitamins A, B_6, B_{12}, C, D, and E. I know those gummies are all the rage these days, but only take them if they are sugar-free and don't have any added artificial flavors or preservatives. I've seen so many that are covered in sugar. A multivitamin isn't supposed to be candy. Finally, be sure to check the expiration date (multivitamins expire, so don't buy something rancid!).

2. **FISH OIL.** Also known as omega-3s, fish oil is one of the nutrients most of us don't get enough of, which is why we need to supplement. Fish oil reduces inflammation,

lowers triglycerides, and boosts the immune system. I prefer fish oil labeled "burpless" or "burp-free" to avoid the bad fish breath or aftertaste. You can also find a multivitamin that has omega-3 added to it, so you don't have to buy and take two separate pills.

3. **VITAMIN D.** Vitamin D is another one of those things most men and women don't get enough of through their food. It helps maintain strong bones, and it's normally something you get when you spend a lot of time in the sun. I'm always trying to stay out of the sun to keep my skin youthful, so I need to get it elsewhere. Specifically, look for vitamin D_3.

4. **VITAMIN B_{12}.** B_{12} vitamin shots are all the rage these days. Lots of health food stores offer an injection of the stuff and promise it will help you fight off sickness and give you an energy boost. A quick shot in the butt gets in the bloodstream a bit quicker than the pill version. Whenever I feel myself getting sick, I get a shot, but I also make sure to take it in pill form daily. It's known to help with the metabolic utilization of fats and protein, which is important on the Super Carb Diet.

5. **VITAMIN C.** Most people think of orange juice when they think of vitamin C. Unfortunately, we can't load up on juice while doing the Super Carb Diet, so supplements are key. Vitamin C is fantastic for the immune system because it fights off infections, colds, and disease.

6. **MAGNESIUM.** This is the supplement I find most people don't take and everyone should. Magnesium deficiency is often caused by heavy exercise or lots of stress,

so chances are a lot of you are deficient. Magnesium is needed to produce and store energy, as well as support regular blood sugar levels. You can take it in pill form, or there's a wonderful variety of flavored powders that are available to take before bed. Mix a little with some hot water and you will sleep like a baby, all the while helping your system work better while you are asleep. I'll also let you in on a little secret that is against some of our rules, but it goes great with magnesium: tart cherry juice (make sure it's JUST tart cherry juice, with nothing added). If you mix a little with your magnesium powder, you will sleep great! You're probably wondering if you need to calculate the tart cherry juice into your daily totals . . . no. This is the one exception. That does NOT mean you can have a bottle of juice every night. It means you can have a SHOT of tart cherry juice with your magnesium before bed. Please make sure you buy the right juice, and do not exceed the limit. Don't drink any ol' juice from the supermarket. I don't want you all drinking a glass of orange juice before bed as a replacement. Specifically, tart cherry juice. Not cherry juice cocktail or apple juice. One shot. That's it. It's TART CHERRY JUICE or nothing.

7. **MELATONIN.** If the magnesium mixed with tart cherry juice isn't doing the trick, melatonin should. This is the sleeping supplement. I want you all to be sleeping seven to nine hours on the Super Carb Diet, and if you have trouble, melatonin will be helpful. I'd prefer you don't take it every night, but it's great for when you want a solid sleep or an earlier bedtime. Plus, it's a

great alternative to those prescription sleep aids. Too many people are taking those drugs to sleep. Many of you may need them, but I urge you to try natural supplements before asking the doctor to prescribe you with medication to help you sleep.

These are the supplements I take daily. The vitamins and minerals will ensure your body has what it needs to work as best as possible on your ninety-day journey and beyond. I know vitamins and supplements are an added expense, but they are very important for your overall health. If you absolutely cannot either afford these, or if you're one of those people that has a hard time taking pills, I want to stress that you should at the very least be taking a multivitamin daily. I've found that as I've gotten older, my body has needed more vitamins and supplements to keep it working. I'm always asking my doctor what I could or should be taking to ensure perfect health. It seems the older we get, the more pills we need to take. Which is a perfect segue into my next topic.

13.

AGING

B ook 'em, Danno, I'm five-oh!" Have you all seen the *SNL* character that Molly Shannon plays? Her name is Sally O'Malley, and she's constantly reminding people she's fifty years old. In my head, that character is loosely based on me. Ever since I turned fifty, I can't stop reminding people how old I am. I wear it like a badge of honor. I'm fifty! Well, now I'm technically fifty-one, but the sentiment remains the same. I'm a survivor and I'll never forget that. A lot of people think that getting older means it's impossible to get the body you want. I'm living proof that that's not true. Sure, there are things that happen to the body that make it more challenging as you age, but it's not quite as cut-and-dried as you think.

After forty-five, the average person loses right around 10 percent of muscle mass per decade.[1] The muscle mass that is lost turns into fat on the body, meaning it's that much harder to get those biceps pumped the way you can in your twenties. We know that muscle burns more calories than fat, which means the body requires fewer calories as we get older. I think back on how much junk food I could eat when I was younger without gaining weight. Now, I can't be so careless. If I want to have a youthful body that lasts through my twilight years, I need to be diligent. And you do, too. Of course, you're not all in your fifties like me. Because of that, I wanted to talk about aging because the body is drastically different throughout the different stages of your life. For those of you that are younger, learn from me. For those of you that are older, do not give up on achieving your goals. Amazing things are possible at any age; you just need to be smart and work hard.

YOUTH/TEENS

Move! It's simple. I was fortunate enough to work with former first lady Michelle Obama on the Let's Move! campaign. The goal was to fight childhood obesity by getting kids to move. When you're a kid and in your teens, your body will want to stay thin, but you must give it something to work with. That means moving. One in five children aged six to nineteen is obese. This number is more than triple what it was in the 1970s.[2] This is too high. I know there probably aren't a lot of fourth graders reading this book, but I'm certain there are a lot of parents of fourth graders reading. People ask me all the time how to help their kids lose weight. It's a problem and we need to fix it. How? First, you need to make sure the kids are eating healthy. I know not every school is offering a well-balanced meal, and even if they are, kids take their lunch money and spend it at the vending machines instead of on the good stuff. Start cooking! Pack their lunches, and have a balanced meal ready for dinner. Make sure they are getting enough sleep so they can make good food decisions. Know that as a parent, it's up to you to put in the work early so that your children have the skills necessary to lead a healthy lifestyle when they leave the nest. Lead by example and cook meals with the same foods we talk about on the Super Carb Diet. And make sure the children are active and that they are moving. Some kids aren't into sports, and that's fine. But they need to run around and find some activity that is going to get their heart rates up. At this age, it's less about the children's choices, and more about the parent's choices.

TWENTIES

The twenties are all about forming habits that will be with you for the rest of your life. Most people are finishing school and settling into their careers in their twenties. This is a huge change, from a lifestyle where people (parents, teachers) were telling you what to do to a lifestyle where you have the freedom to make your own choices. Your body is still working in your favor in your twenties. In fact, you build bone until roughly age twenty-five, and when the body is building bone, it's burning extra calories without your even doing a thing. You can still get away with eating junk and exercising sparingly in your twenties, but it will all catch up with you in your thirties. That's why you should focus on creating healthy habits at this stage of your life. If you're reading this in your twenties, don't let your eating get out of control after you leave college. You assume the weight will be easy to get off, so you just keep eating and eating. I see it all the time. Then you reach your thirties with extra weight that won't come off as easy as it once did. Don't let this happen to you.

Your twenties are also a time to experiment with fitness. You're no longer playing in sports leagues that your parents signed you up for, or getting a free gym membership on your college campus. That means you must seek a workout on your own. Going to the gym is another habit you need to form in your twenties because it will be much harder to develop that habit in your thirties or forties. People are often obese in their forties and fifties simply because they didn't make these lifestyle choices in their twenties and they're scared of the unknown. They've never been to a gym before, so the idea of joining one later in life becomes terrifying to them and, in turn, they can't lose the weight. I don't want you to have to worry about that down the road. Put in the work now. To all my twenty-somethings out there, just know that the choices you make right now are going to stick with you.

THIRTIES

The thirties are all about adding weight lifting to your regimen if you haven't already. Like I said earlier, your muscle mass declines drastically in your forties, but it starts its descent in your thirties. To combat this loss, it's important to start strength training. Look, the treadmill is great for a sweat, but your body needs more, particularly as you start aging. I'm not a runner anymore, but I see the benefits. However, grabbing a barbell and lifting it is going to do wonders for your body. Hopefully you have developed a routine of going to the gym multiple times a week by the time you reach your thirties. That's the time to start targeting your body. If you start weight lifting in your thirties, you'll be that much better off when muscle decline starts to happen even more rapidly in your forties. Start small and grow. Don't be intimidated by the weight room. Even those muscle guys you see deadlifting four hundred pounds had to start somewhere. Also, start moisturizing in your thirties and using sunscreen if you haven't already. You know what? Do that no matter what age group you fall in. Right now. Every day. Sunscreen is everything.

FORTIES

Ah, the forties. I think of them as the plateau years. Your body isn't working quite like it used to. You won't get the same results you once did. What I mean is, it won't be as easy to get your biceps to pop or to get those model abs. This causes frustration and a weight plateau. You get in a rut. And you need to get out of it so you successfully get out of your forties alive. That means you need, once again, to alter your workout routine. I don't just mean changing the movements you're doing at the gym. I mean you may have to change scenery. I love the gym I go to, but I also travel a lot. This keeps things feeling fresh for me. When I'm out of town, I always find a facility I can use, and when I'm living in New York or LA, I am constantly trying new classes and experimenting with every new fitness craze that comes along. I encourage you to do the same. There are SO many options out there, so don't get stuck at a place you hate.

A lot of people tell me about the beautiful home gyms they set up on their quest to get fit. They load their basements with expensive equipment so they can work out whenever they please. While it's great to have a home gym, it's not for everyone. Oftentimes I find clients and friends get restless working out in the confines of their own home. It's lonely. There's no eye candy to keep you motivated. Just because you have enough money to set up a weight bench and treadmill in your home doesn't mean you should. Sometimes spending fifty dollars a month to go to a gym nearby is going to be more beneficial in the long run. It will take you outside your comfort zone, and seeing other people working out will open your eyes to new movements and options for exercise. Plus, it's a great opportunity to socialize. Some of my best friends are people that I met at my gym. It's an immediate shared interest, and you always have something to do together. By the time you reach your forties, it's harder than ever to make new friends and meet new people. I encourage you to find a gym and do just that.

FIFTIES

Fifty is the time to be fabulous! Granted, I'm biased because I'm currently fifty-one, but I truly believe fifty is when you hit your stride. You know what you like and what you don't like when it comes to food and fitness. You've lived with your body long enough to know your problem areas. Unfortunately, your fifties are also when your hormones start to go wild. For women, I'm talking menopause. According to the North American Menopause Society, the average age of women experiencing menopause is fifty-one.[3] Of course, that varies anywhere from forties to sixties, but it gives you a rough idea of what you have in store for your fifties. There's hot flashes and exhaustion. Your body is changing.

It's not just women, either. Men experience a hormonal shift in their fifties as well. Granted, the change is not quite as intense as for women, but it happens. Working out consistently is going to help you when these bodily changes take place. It will keep the endorphins flowing when your mood is all over the place.

When you reach your fifties, you must start buckling down and getting strict about your diet and exercise. You don't have a choice. If you want to live to see your sixties, seventies, and eighties, it's crucial. My heart attack was a brutal reminder that I need to continue to take care of myself, just like all of you. If I wasn't as healthy as I am, I might not have survived, let alone recovered so quickly. Like I said, I'm a survivor and I've truly never felt better. For those of you approaching your fifties and worried it's all downhill, take it from me: I've never looked or felt better than I do right now. I know that sounds vain, but it's true. Look back at some old episodes of *The Biggest Loser* and tell me you don't agree. I've aged well because I take care of myself, and it's never too late to start! Aside from my physical health, I've learned to let go of the small things. I don't sweat the small stuff, and that's one of the wonderful benefits of getting older.

SIXTIES AND BEYOND

Okay, so I haven't quite gotten to this age yet, but I do know a thing or two about this time in your life. Obviously, the staples of the Super Carb Diet still apply: diet, exercise, and sleep. You can still work out and be active. Aging is no excuse to stop going to the gym and trying new things. Other than that, it's time to start focusing on mental exercises. You must keep your mind active. Keeping your brain sharp is going to be so important going forward. Read. Do a crossword puzzle. Play Tetris. Watch *Jeopardy!* Work your brain out.

Aging is scary for a lot of people. Your body and mind change so drastically as you get older, which makes it even more important to remain diligent with everything you've learned on the Super Carb Diet. If you're young, you have all the time in the world to get healthy, but your body is waiting for you to make the commitment. The longer you wait, the harder it will be. For those of you that are older, focus and get to work. I'm not going to lie, it's going to be harder to get the body you want as you age. But amazing things are possible if you work hard. Don't give up simply because of the number of candles on your birthday cake. Put the work in and you'll feel like a kid again!

14.

SCALING

I mentioned you're going to have to do all your own cooking on the Super Carb Diet, right? Cooking is the only way to know *exactly* what's going in your food. This means spending a lot of time in your kitchen. And I want you to get a food scale. It's going to keep you accountable. Unfortunately, most people aren't familiar with food scales, so I'm here to break it down. There are two main types of food scales:

1. Digital
2. Balance

The digital scale is ideal for this diet. It's going to be more accurate and quicker than the balance scales out there. Digital scales used to be more expensive, but nowadays you can get them for under thirty dollars from most places, in-store and online. What do I look for? One with easy-to-read numbers. If you see me around town, you'll notice I usually simultaneously have a pair of reading glasses on my face, on my head, and in my bag. My eyes aren't the best, so I use a food scale with a large digital display. There are also great options for scales with cups or bowls attached so you can throw your food right in and not worry about dirtying an extra dish.

To measure your food, you need to zero out your scale between each ingredient. For most digital scales, it will already be zeroed out when you turn it on; just make sure nothing is placed on top of it. If your scale does not come with a bowl attached, you will need to weigh your container or plate without the food on it so you can subtract that number. I know, I know, I'm giving you more math. Deal. You then put your food on the plate, place it on the scale, subtract the weight of the plate, and voilà! You have your measurements.

You may be wondering when to weigh your food—before or after cooking. If so, good! You're using your brain. Some foods weigh less after cooking than before, so when should you put them on the scale?

MEAT: BEFORE cooking when possible

EVERYTHING ELSE: BEFORE cooking

Basically that means everything should be weighed before cooking, and that's true, but I wanted to separate the two categories because it's not always possible to weigh meat before cooking. I prefer that you weigh it raw because nutrition labels correspond with the raw version of the meat. When you cook it, the moisture in the meat evaporates, so it weighs less. Unfortunately, you won't always be working with raw meat. If you purchase a grilled chicken breast from the grocery store, or a ready-to-eat rotisserie chicken to use in one of your recipes to save some time, you'll be working with cooked meat instead of raw. There are ways to get a more accurate measurement when you're dealing with these cooked meats, but it's very complicated and we want to simplify scaling as much as possible. So, when you're cooking meat, do your best to measure BEFORE you start cooking. It will give you a more accurate reading for the nutritional value of your meal.

If you don't have a food scale handy (perhaps you're cooking at a friend's house or your current scale is broken), there are some ways to work around this situation. It's not going to be as accurate as a scale, but you can make do. Here are the basics:

3 ounces of meat=a deck of cards or the palm of your hand

1 slice of bread=a cassette tape

½ cup of cooked rice, pasta, or fruit=½ baseball

These numbers aren't exact, but they will work in a pinch. You're probably thinking, "One slice of bread can't possibly be the size of a cassette tape; that seems small." You're right! A slice of bread shouldn't be much bigger than that. However, lots of breads out there are huge. That's why we need a food scale. So many foods are bigger than they should be, so we have no concept of proper serving sizes anymore. Everything is made bigger in the United States and the proportions are screwing up our bodies. Working with a food scale and calculating your numbers are going to show you just how off your brain is when it comes to measuring food. You will see times when you think you aren't eating much, you actually are eating a lot. The Super Carb Diet is going to retrain your brain to look at food and find out how much is supposed to be eaten, instead of how much food companies have told us to eat. Eventually, you won't need a scale. When you weigh chicken four or five times a week, you will start to understand how much it weighs just by looking at it. This goes back to why I don't want you eating in restaurants for the ninety days you are doing the Super Carb Diet. Even when you can have something like a chicken breast cooked without oil or other sauces, most people still don't understand serving sizes. By the end of your ninety days, you will be able to go to a restaurant and look at a grilled chicken breast and know exactly how much to eat to stay within your numbers. That goes for everything, not just meat.

One of my friends recently got on the Super Carb Diet and told me that one of the things he noticed immediately was how he was miscalculating the amount of skim milk he added to his coffee. He said for years he would use one of those flavored creamers and eyeball the amount every morning, assuming it was about one tablespoon. When he switched to skim milk and began measuring everything, he realized that he was using about four tablespoons of creamer in his coffee every morning. This is especially substantial when dealing with something like artificially flavored creamer that is high in calories, sugar, and artificial ingredients. He was drinking lots of calories before even getting to his meal in the morning. Once he started using an actual tablespoon, he saw the difference. That's why it's crucial you start to measure all the foods that are going into your body. Eventually, you won't need to weigh the food, because you'll be smart enough to know the answers. The ninety days are training you for the rest of your life.

15.

DEAR DIARY

I like organization—in my life, in my diet, and in my workouts. The Super Carb Diet is all about organization, and I want to make it as easy as possible for you to adhere to my plan. By now, you know the rules. You have your numbers, the foods you can and cannot eat, and the other rules to follow to be successful. Now you just need to organize all your info. The ninety days will be much easier if you start with organization. I use a journal. You can write all your info into your phone for easy access, or on one of those whiteboards that go on your refrigerator. Whatever works best for you, I support, as long as you are organized. This may seem like an unimportant step, but it's not. How you keep track of your daily activity is going to make a huge difference in the long run.

Earlier, I had you write down all your numbers on a piece of paper. You probably just grabbed whatever scrap or piece of loose-leaf that was near you at the time. That's okay, but now I want you to be deliberate. Hop on your computer or open a blank notebook that you can use for the next ninety days. When I first started the Super Carb Diet, I printed out ninety pages (sample on pages 146–147), to keep track of my daily numbers. Each day I posted a new sheet on my refrigerator. It became my food journal. Again, you can do this on one of those whiteboards and just erase every day (although it's good to keep your journal beyond the ninety days, which I'll go into later), or you can keep track on your phone or through one of the many apps that count calories, carbs, protein, and fat. Which-ever method you choose, I want you to do this every day. There's a lot you need to keep track of, and all the numbers will get all mixed up unless you have a system in place. With my journal, I broke down each day by meal, and listed the carbs, protein, and fat I ate at each meal. I left some space to do my math and any adding I needed.

On the bottom of each page, I put some space to write in how much sleep I got the night before. Keeping track of the hours I slept helped me to understand how sleep affected me throughout the diet. On the days I got less than seven hours of sleep the night prior, I noticed my workouts were harder to get through and my diet was harder to plan. My focus wasn't as sharp as the days following the proper amount of sleep.

I included a sample of one of my daily journals here in this book. You'll see that I added spots for my weight, my waist, and my work-out. Again, some days your weight will fluctuate even if you are adhering to the rules. Water weight is a tricky thing, so don't get discouraged if you go up or down a pound within a few days. Writing down your weight every day will, however, give you a good idea of your progress over the duration of the ninety days. Day 1 will look very different from day 90.

Your waist size is not something you need to measure every day. I measure mine once a week, but you can measure it once every other week if you prefer. If you decide to measure it once a week, be sure to do it on the same day each week and mark it in your journal. The idea is for you to track all your progress. You'll see in my journal that I also left a space for my workout. My workouts are consistent at CrossFit, so I typically just checked off to note that I worked out for the day. If I did something different, I would make note of it. If you are new to the gym, you can leave a little extra space and write down what you did for your workout each day. Then you will be able to track your strength and progress in the gym over the entire ninety days.

I know it's a pain in the ass to print out ninety sheets of paper, but I also know it will help keep you on track. I find that printing out my customized food journal is the best method for success. You may find something totally different that works for you. You can buy a food journal from the store and customize it with our rules, or you can use one of those handy apps on your phone. A lot of those apps will even tell you the number of carbs, protein, and fat in the foods you're eating, WHILE adding the numbers for you. Technology makes it easier than ever to lose weight. If you're using one of those apps, be sure it is accurate. Sometimes they have a lot of different options for a specific food and you end up choosing the wrong one, which will throw you off. Not only do I want you to be certain you are inputting the right foods, I want you to double-check the serving size each time. If you don't have a smartphone, or like me, prefer to use paper and pen, I recommend creating a journal like mine and posting it each day on the refrigerator to keep track. Here's what mine looks like:

DAY 1

BREAKFAST

Carbs:

Protein:

Fat:

Vegetable:

NOTES
_____

LUNCH

Carbs:

Protein:

Fat:

Vegetable:

NOTES
_____

DINNER

Carbs:

Protein:

Fat:

Vegetable:

NOTES
_____

FLOATER

Protein:

Fat:

NOTES
_____

| WEIGHT | WAIST | SLEEP | WORKOUT |

In the next chapter, I'll show you what a typical menu looks like for a 185-pound male, but for now I want you to create a similar workbook for yourself. You can go to the nearest office supply store and photocopy the sheet right from this book, or simply create something similar using your blank notebook/computer. Whatever method you choose, be sure to have your workbook ready before the next day starts. Every night get the next day's journal prepared. If you are planning on using one of those apps, log onto your phone right now, download the food journal app of choice and play around with it. Understand how it works before you start the diet. I don't care which method you choose, I only care that you are keeping yourself accountable every single day. We all lead busy lives, so this little step will save you just a little time each day. That little time will help immensely. Trust me.

16.

SUPER CARB DIET
FOR BEGINNERS

You got the book. You did the reading. Now all you need to do is start the diet. It's overwhelming. It's ESPECIALLY overwhelming if you've never dieted before, or if you've never read a nutrition label in your life. Or if you can't do math. I can't do math, so I was overwhelmed at first, too. But I pushed my way through it, because if I learned anything from *The Devil Wears Prada,* it's that you must put in the work to get the outcome you want. I also learned that Meryl looks great with a white wig. And that Anne's friends in that movie were assholes. That doesn't have much to do with this diet, but it's important. Always surround yourself with good people. You'll have a better success rate with everything you do.

Up until now this whole thing has been a lot of those numbers, and science, and facts. Don't think I don't see it, I do. And numbers are scary. And science is confusing. And facts are overwhelming! The thought of calculating everything you eat and keeping track of all the good foods and bad foods is . . . well, it's a lot. I told you it would be worth it in the end, but I just can't shake the thought of you all reading and getting scared. I've seen it happen before. People get overwhelmed by everything it takes to lose weight and make changes to your body. I don't want you to be deterred from the Super Carb Diet because I know it has the power to change your life. I've seen the results in my own body, and I've seen the results in friends I've shared this plan with. The problem is those numbers and rules are a lot to take in. Most of you probably stopped doing math like that in high school. I know I did. But like I said, the work you put in is going to directly affect the results you see down the line. The numbers are going to come easy to you later, but until they do, I want you to know that this is doable, and you are going to be able to eat normal meals. Delicious, even. This isn't a diet where you will starve yourself, and it's not going to suck the fun out of the food. You get to eat. A lot. And the foods you're allowed to eat are fantastic. You don't have to eat a plain plate of lettuce every meal. Your plate is going to have everything you need, and it will be satisfying.

For beginners, I've laid out fourteen days (!) of meals for you to start your diet. That's two weeks! You can start here, or you can do your own thing, as long as you stay within your numbers. That means women should be having the amount or protein they calculated, 30 grams of carbs, and 12 grams of fat for these meals, while men should have the amount of protein they calculated, 40 grams of carbs, and 15 grams of fat. Plus, you can have those 75 extra calories of veggies. Once you hit your carb, protein, and fat numbers, you can add in 75 extra calories of veggies. That means you can eat them as a side dish, or add some extras into your recipes. Monitor your grocery lists accordingly. These fourteen days lay out the basics, but they aren't recipes. They are suggestions to help you plan your meals for the first two weeks. There are recipes in the back of the book, but these sample days keep things easy for people who have never been fans of cooking. I tried to give you basic suggestions (sandwiches, lots of chicken and eggs) to get started and slowly ease you into the more time-consuming recipes. I've also included seven days of a sample men's food journal so you can see exactly what that looks like with the numbers included. I don't know how to make it any easier for all of you. You can even rip this chapter out and take it to the grocery store to do your shopping. I excluded nutrition facts on purpose. You'll need to craft these meals to fit your own Super Carb plate. That means your side salad might have some olives or seeds, or your chicken breast might be bigger or smaller, depending on your current size and numbers. Adjust accordingly.

14-DAY SAMPLE MENU

DAY 1

BREAKFAST

Carb: 100% whole grain muffin

Protein: Egg whites

Fat: Avocado, oil

Vegetable: Spinach

Cooking: Use a nonstick pan with 1–2 seconds of olive oil cooking spray to cook your egg whites. I like to scramble with the spinach and then add to a toasted whole grain muffin and top with some avocado. Note: Just because it says avocado, it does NOT mean a whole avocado. A little goes a long way, so make sure you aren't eating an entire one for these meals. Quite honestly, you should never be eating a whole avocado. A little dab will do ya.

LUNCH

Carb: Cauliflower, carrots, and broccoli mix

Protein: Chicken breast

Fat: Slivered almonds, oil

Vegetable: Broccoli mix

Cooking: This meal is super quick and delicious. Grill the chicken breast or sauté in a little bit of oil. Roast the veggies along with the slivered almonds and season with your favorite spices.

DINNER

Carb: 100% Whole-grain bun

Protein: Lean ground chicken burger

Fat: Side salad with balsamic vinegar/oil dressing

Vegetable: Extra-big salad

Cooking: Grill the ground chicken patty and put on the whole-grain bun. Finish the meal with a side salad using your own dressing. For the dressing, simply mix oil and vinegar with some lemon juice, salt, and pepper. Men should be having 1 tablespoon of oil for the dressing, while women should have no more than 1½ teaspoons of olive oil. If you have some fat grams left over, you can add some avocado to your side salad or mash it up and top your burger with it.

FLOATER

Protein: Nonfat Greek yogurt

Fat: ½ tablespoon nut butter

DAY 2

BREAKFAST

Carb: 100% Whole-grain toast

Protein: Nonfat Greek yogurt

Fat: Crushed almonds

Vegetable: Red bell peppers, raw

Cooking: Throw the almonds in the yogurt and eat separately or spread it on the toast and enjoy!

LUNCH

Carb: 100 % Whole-wheat wrap, chopped peppers

Protein: Lean ground chicken

Fat: Avocado

Vegetable: Red bell peppers

Cooking: Roast red peppers and sauté ground chicken. Eat as a burrito.

DINNER

Carb: 100% Whole-wheat tortilla, grilled peppers and onions, salsa

Protein: Grilled chicken breast

Fat: Avocado

Vegetable: Grilled banana peppers

Cooking: Add some salsa and use grilled chicken instead of ground chicken to change things up from your lunch.

FLOATER

Protein: Egg white protein shake

DAY 3

BREAKFAST

Carb: Steel-cut oats

Protein: Egg whites

Fat: Egg yolks

Vegetable: Spinach

Cooking: I don't always eat a whole egg; usually I just use the egg whites, but for this breakfast, use the yolks as your fat.

LUNCH

Carbs: Brown rice, chopped lettuce, tomatoes, and onions

Protein: Grilled chicken

Fat: Guacamole

Vegetable: Side salad

Cooking: Mix ingredients and eat as a bowl.

DINNER

Carb: Roasted Brussels sprouts

Protein: Grilled halibut

Fat: Oil

Vegetable: Brussels sprouts

Cooking: Use olive oil as your fat and top the halibut and Brussels sprouts with it to add some flavor and moisture.

FLOATER

Protein: Canned white-meat tuna in water

DAY 4

BREAKFAST

Carb: Orange, 100% Whole-grain toast

Protein: Egg whites

Fat: Peanut butter

Vegetable: Spinach

Cooking: Toast the bread and cook the egg whites. For the peanut butter, I would simply scoop a teaspoon or so to finish off the meal and give the breakfast a little extra oomph.

LUNCH

Carb: Banana

Protein: Zero-carb whey protein

Fat: Almond butter

Vegetable: Kale

Cooking: Blend ingredients and drink your lunch.

DINNER

Carb: Wild rice, asparagus

Protein: Grilled chicken breast

Fat: Oil

Vegetable: Asparagus

Cooking: Use the olive oil in the cooking, and/or add to the final product for some extra flavor.

FLOATER

Protein: Leftover grilled chicken breast

DAY 5

BREAKFAST

Carb: 100% Whole-grain toast

Protein: Egg whites

Fat: Avocado

Vegetable: Bell peppers, raw

Cooking: Toast the bread and enjoy as a sandwich.

LUNCH

Protein/Carb/Fat: Italian Wedding Soup (see page 262)

Vegetable: Added extra vegetables for a heartier soup

DINNER

Carb: 100% Whole-grain tortilla

Protein: Grilled chicken

Fat: Kalamata olives, feta cheese

Vegetable: Side salad

Cooking: Top the grilled chicken with the lettuce, olives, and feta cheese to give it a Greek flair.

FLOATER

Protein: Deli turkey

Fat: Walnuts

DAY 6

BREAKFAST

Protein/Carb/Fat: Protein Pancakes (see page 255)

Vegetable: Bell peppers, raw

LUNCH

Carb: Banana

Protein: Egg white protein powder

Fat: Almond butter

Vegetable: Roasted green beans

Cooking: Blend the ingredients for a liquid lunch.

DINNER

Carbs/Fat: Persian cucumber salad

Protein: Grilled chicken breast

Vegetable: Asparagus

Cooking: Add grilled chicken to a Persian Cucumber Salad.

FLOATER

Protein: Leftover grilled chicken breast

DAY 7

BREAKFAST

Carb: Banana

Protein: Egg whites

Fat: Peanut butter

Vegetable: Roasted okra

Cooking: Slice the banana sideways and spread a little peanut butter on top for a delicious treat! Okra also makes a great side.

LUNCH

Protein/Carb/Fat: Chicken Meatballs (see page 245) with brown rice

Vegetable: Roasted broccoli

Cooking: Top the brown rice with the ground chicken meatballs.

DINNER

Carb: Zucchini noodles

Protein/Fat: Chicken Meatballs (see Lunch menu)

Vegetable: Side salad

Cooking: Eat the ground chicken meatballs on cooked zucchini noodles for a change from lunch.

FLOATER

None.

BREAKFAST

Carb: Steel-cut oats

Protein: Nonfat plain Greek yogurt

Fat: Almonds

Vegetable: Bell peppers, raw

Cooking: Mix what you can here. Depending on your numbers, you may have to forgo some of the yogurt for the oats or almonds. Work with what you have.

LUNCH

Carb: Tortilla, salsa

Protein: Mahi-mahi

Fat: Olive oil

Vegetable: Romaine lettuce

Cooking: Mahi-mahi tacos are delicious. Use the olive oil to cook the fish. Top with lots of romaine.

DINNER

Protein/Carb/Fat: Cauliflower "Fried" Rice (see page 250) with lean ground turkey

Vegetable: Side salad

FLOATER

Protein: Lean ground turkey

Fat: Olive oil

Cooking: Top some cooked ground turkey with a little olive oil to add flavor.

BREAKFAST

Carb: Apple

Protein: Egg white protein powder

Fat: Peanut butter

Vegetable: Celery, raw

Cooking: Mix the protein powder in some water. Dip the apples and celery in the peanut butter.

LUNCH

Carb: Banana

Protein: Protein powder

Fat: Almond butter

Vegetable: Kale

Cooking: Blend ingredients together with some ice and make a smoothie.

DINNER

Carb: Sweet potato

Protein/Fat: Filet mignon

Vegetable: Spinach

Cooking: The filet mignon is a lean cut of meat, but it still has fat, so it is going to count as your protein and fat for the meal. I don't recommend red meat often, but it's okay every once in a while (unless your doctor advises you otherwise).

FLOATER

Protein/Fat: Leftover filet mignon

BREAKFAST

Carb: 1 slice 100% Whole-grain bread, toasted

Protein: Egg whites

Fat: Avocado

Vegetable: Bell peppers

Cooking: Mix the egg whites and peppers together to make an omelet and top with avocado.

LUNCH

Carb: Romaine lettuce, peppercinis (banana peppers)

Protein: Grilled chicken

Fat: Olive oil, green olives

Vegetable: This is a super-sized salad

Cooking: Make a salad and mix your favorite greens with some olive oil dressing and olives as your fat.

DINNER

Protein/Carb/Fat/Vegetable: Ground Chicken Bolognese (see page 260)

FLOATER

Protein: Deli turkey slice

Fat: Walnuts

BREAKFAST

Carb: 1 slice of 100% Whole-grain bread, toasted

Protein/Fat: Protein Pancakes (see page 255)

Vegetable: Carrots

Cooking: Make the recipe and if you have leftover carbs, have a small piece of the bread you bought earlier. Carrots make a great side.

LUNCH

Carb/Fat/Vegetable: Rice and Kale Moroccan Salad (see page 259)

Protein: Protein powder

Cooking: This is a veggie lunch. Use a veggie protein powder and mix with water, then cook the rice and kale Moroccan salad recipe.

DINNER

Protein/Carb/Fat: Tofu

Vegetable: Roasted broccoli and carrots

Cooking: Tofu is great for a vegetarian meal. It's got protein, carbs, and fat, so serve with some veggies like roasted broccoli and carrots.

FLOATER

Fat: Almonds

BREAKFAST

Carb: 1 slice of 100% Whole-grain bread, toasted

Protein: Nonfat plain Greek yogurt

Fat: Peanut butter

Vegetable: Celery

Cooking: Top the bread with peanut butter. Celery on the side.

LUNCH

Carb: Brown rice

Protein: Sautéed chicken breast

Fat: Olive oil

Vegetable: Persian Cucumber Salad

Cooking: Sauté chicken in olive oil.

DINNER

Protein/Carb/Fat/Vegetable: Chicken Burrito (see page 256)

FLOATER

Protein: Egg white protein shake

Cooking: Mix with water or almond milk for your floater meal.

BREAKFAST

Carb: Tortilla/salsa

Protein: Egg whites

Fat: Avocado

Vegetable: Spinach

Cooking: Use a low-carb tortilla to make a breakfast burrito with your egg whites and spinach.

LUNCH

Carb: Tortilla

Protein/Fat: Bison Tacos (see page 253)

Vegetable: Side salad

Cooking: Using the bison taco recipe, have a low-carb tortilla as your shell instead of the lettuce.

DINNER

Protein/Carb/Fat/Vegetable: Feta Olive Wrap (see page 249)

FLOATER

Protein: Deli turkey

DAY 14

BREAKFAST

Carb: 100% Whole-grain English muffin

Protein/Fat: Protein Pancakes (see page 255)

Cooking: Depending on your numbers, you may not have room on your plate for the English muffin. That's okay! The protein pancakes are filling.

LUNCH

Protein/Carb/Fat/Vegetable: Lemon Pepper Bowl (see page 248)

DINNER

Protein/Carb/Fat: Slow Cooker Turkey Chili (see page 247)

Vegetable: Side salad

FLOATER

Protein: Canned white meat tuna

Now that you have a blueprint for the first two weeks, I want you to see how to craft your plate to fit within your numbers. Again, every journal is going to look different based on your tastes, numbers, and habits. You can plan your weeks like the following sample journal for a man at 180 pounds, or you can find foods that work for you. I did this so you can see how well-rounded and diverse these meals are, but remember that I'm barely scratching the surface on what you can make to eat. You can see exactly how the meals fit within the numbers for a typical 180-pound man. For some meals it's the exact amount of carbs, protein, and fat allotted, while for other meals it's a little bit less. Those 75 extra calories of veggies are ON TOP OF the rest of your numbers, so you'll see in the following food journal that they aren't incorporated into the TOTAL numbers. Get it? Those extra veggies are to fill you up and satiate. Sometimes those vegetables will be incorporated into the recipe, and sometimes you'll eat those on the side. Hopefully the sample journal gives you a good idea of what you can do with your days. I also included some notes for each day so you can get an idea of what went on behind the madness.

SAMPLE FOOD JOURNAL

BREAKFAST

Coffee, black (0 g Carbs, 0 g Protein, 0 g Fat)

2 slices toasted sunflower bread (30 g Carbs, 6 g Protein, 4 g Fat)

Nonfat plain Greek yogurt (7 g Carbs, 18 g Protein, 0 g Fat)

1 tablespoon peanut butter (3 g Carbs, 4 g Protein, 8 g Fat)

Vegetable: 1½ cups roasted brussels sprouts

TOTAL: 40 g Carbs, 28 g Protein, 14 g Fat

LUNCH

Tortilla (24 g Carbs, 6 g Protein, 4 g Fat)

1 cup egg whites, cooked (0 g Carbs, 20 g Protein, 0 g Fat)

2 oz. salsa (4 g Carbs, 2 g Protein, 0 g Fat)

1 cup cauliflower (5 g Carbs, 2 g Protein, 0 g Fat)

2 oz. avocado (4 g Carbs, 2 g Protein, 8 g Fat)

Vegetable: 5 cups spinach, cooked

TOTAL: 37 g Carbs, 32 g Protein, 12 g Fat

DINNER

4 oz. Lean ground chicken breast (1 g Carbs, 26 g Protein, 1 g Fat)

⅜ cup brown rice (33 g Carbs, 0 g Protein, 3 g Fat)

2 oz. avocado (4 g Carbs, 2 g Protein, 8 g Fat)

Vegetable: 2 cups roasted asparagus

TOTAL: 38 g Carbs, 28 g Protein, 12 g Fat

FLOATER MEAL

4 oz. Deli turkey meat (0 g Carbs, 22 g Protein, 1 g Fat)

TOTAL: 0 g Carbs, 22 g Protein, 1 g Fat

Takeaways: This breakfast was under the allotted macronutrients for the day. When I'm trying to lose weight, I find breakfast to be the easiest place to lower my food intake. I'm usually not craving much when I first wake up, so I like to think of breakfast as my fuel meal, meaning I get what I need to get the day going, but I don't indulge in extras.

DAY 2

BREAKFAST

Coffee, black (0 g Carbs, 0 g Protein, 0 g Fat)

Egg White Tower Sandwich:

1 cup egg whites, cooked (0 g Carbs, 20 g Protein, 0 g Fat)

2 slices of 100% whole-grain (thin-sliced) bread (26 g Carbs,

6 g Protein, 4 g Fat)

2 oz. avocado (4 g Carbs, 2 g Protein, 8 g Fat)

1.5 oz. salsa (3 g Carbs, 1.5 g Protein, 0 g Fat)

Vegetable: 1 large bell pepper

TOTAL: 33 g Carbs, 29.5 g Protein, 12 g Fat

LUNCH

Chicken meatballs over spaghetti squash:

4 oz. lean ground chicken (0 g Carbs, 22 g Protein, 9 g Fat)

¼ egg (0 g Carbs, 1.5 g Protein, 1.25 g Fat)

½ tablespoon milled flaxseed (1 g Carbs, .75 g Protein, 1 g Fat)

¼ tablespoon olive oil (0 g Carbs, 0 g Protein, 3.5 g Fat)

2 cups spaghetti squash (14 g Carbs, 2 g Protein, 0 g Fat)

Vegetable: extra spaghetti squash

TOTAL: 15 g Carbs, 26.25 g Protein, 14.75 g Fat

DINNER

Meatless Ground Burrito:

⅓ cup meatless ground (5 g Carbs, 9 g Protein, .5 g Fat)

1 cup broccoli, chopped (6 g Carbs, 3 g Protein, 0 g Fat)

Lettuce (1 g Carbs, 1 g Protein, 0 g Fat)

1.5 oz. salsa (3 g Carbs, 1.5 g Protein, 0 g Fat)

1 tortilla (10 g Carbs, 3 g Protein, 1 g Fat)

2 oz. avocado (4 g Carbs, 2 g Protein, 8 g Fat)

Vegetable: 2 cups air-fried kale chips

TOTAL: 29 g Carbs, 19.5 g Protein, 9.5 g Fat

FLOATER MEAL

1.5 scoops zero-carb whey protein isolate (0 g Carbs,

30 g Protein, 1 g Fat)

TOTAL: 0 g Carbs, 30 g Protein, 1 g Fat

Takeaways: Meatballs are so versatile and you can customize them in lots of different ways. I've included one of my favorite meatball recipes in the Recipes section. I'll always make enough for leftovers and eat them throughout the week. Get creative with them. Find a lean ground meat (chicken, turkey) and put it over rice, squash, or zucchini noodles for a faux spaghetti and meatballs. You can even make the Italian Wedding Soup recipe for cold winter nights. If you make enough at the beginning of the week, you can use them a variety of ways for lunches and dinner, or make a carb-free version for your floater meals.

BREAKFAST

Coffee, black (0 g Carbs, 0 g Protein, 0 g Fat)

Greek yogurt with berries, nuts, and toast:

1 container (150 g) nonfat plain Greek yogurt (7 g Carbs, 18 g Protein, 0 g Fat)

1 slice 100% whole-grain toast (14 g Carbs, 4 g Protein, 0.5 g Fat)

1 cup strawberries (11 g Carbs, 1 g Protein, 0 g Fat)

.75 oz. almonds (4 g Carbs, 4.5 g Protein, 10.5 g Fat)

Vegetable: 2 cups air-fried kale chips

TOTAL: 36 g Carbs, 27.5 g Protein, 11 g Fat

LUNCH

1 Mahi-Mahi taco (see page 240) (23 g Carbs, 14 g Protein, 6 g Fat)

Side salad (lettuce, olive oil, vinegar, walnut shavings) (3 g Carbs, 4 g Protein, 3 g Fat)

½ cup garden vegetables, roasted (8 g Carbs, 2 g Protein, 5 g Fat)

Vegetable: 1½ cups extra broccoli

TOTAL: 34 g Carbs, 20 g Protein, 14 g Fat

DINNER

4 oz. grilled chicken breast (0 g Carbs, 25 g Protein, 4 g Fat)

1¼ cups shaved Brussels sprouts (8 g Carbs, 3 g Protein, 0 g Fat)

1 cup cooked brown rice (22 g Carbs, 3 g Protein, 1 g Fat)

Vegetable: 1 cup spinach, cooked

TOTAL: 30 g Carbs, 31 g Protein, 5 g Fat

FLOATER MEAL

2 Zero-Carb deviled eggs (0 g Carbs, 11.4 g Protein, 12.2 g Fat)

TOTAL: 0 g Carbs, 11.4 g Protein, 12.2 g Fat

Takeaways: I LOVE roasting veggies. You can pick one or mix a few different types for a medley. I season before cooking so the flavors soak into the vegetables. Just be sure to go easy on the oil. When I'm cooking with clients, I notice they throw oil on vegetables as if it's water on an open flame. It's too much. You must keep track of the oil you're cooking with, so measure it out by teaspoon before roasting and calculate that into your plate equation. Also, don't be afraid of those olive oil sprays. They are great for limiting your oil intake.

DAY 4

BREAKFAST

Coffee, black (0 g Carbs, 0 g Protein, 0 g Fat)

Ham and Egg Breakfast Burrito:

1 cup egg whites, cooked (0 g Carbs, 20 g Protein, 0 g Fat)

1 oz. ham (1 g Carbs, 5 g Protein, 1 g Fat)

1.5 oz. salsa (3 g Carbs, 1.5 g Protein, 0 g Fat)

1 tortilla (24 g Carbs, 6 g Protein, 3 g Fat)

Vegetable: 1 cup spinach, cooked

TOTAL: 28 g Carbs, 32.5 g Protein, 4 g Fat

LUNCH

Salad:

2 cups butter lettuce (0 g Carbs, 2 g Protein, 0 g Fat)

3 oz. grilled chicken (0 g Carbs, 25.8 g Protein, 3 g Fat)

4.3 oz. pomegranate seeds (20 g Carbs, 2 g Protein, 1 g Fat)

¾ tablespoon olive oil (0 g Carbs, 0 g Protein, 10 g Fat)

1 tablespoon vinegar (0 g Carbs, 0 g Protein, 0 g Fat)

1 tablespoon lemon juice (2 g Carbs, 0 g Protein, 0 g Fat)

Vegetable: Mix in some other lettuces for a super-sized salad

TOTAL: 22 g Carbs, 29.8 g Protein, 14 g Fat

DINNER

Bison Burger with "Fries":

4 oz. ground bison patty (0 g Carbs, 20 g Protein, 11 g Fat)

1 tomato slice (1 g Carbs, 0 g Protein, 0 g Fat)

Romaine lettuce (0 g Carbs, 0 g Protein, 0 g Fat)

1 teaspoon yellow mustard (0 g Carbs, 0 g Protein, 0 g Fat)

2 slices 100% whole-grain bread (28 g Carbs, 8 g Protein, 1 g Fat)

½ cup sweet potato "fries" (13 g Carbs, 1 g Protein, 0 g Fat)

Vegetable: Small side salad

TOTAL: 42 g Carbs, 29 g Protein, 12 g Fat)

FLOATER MEAL

2 slices deli turkey (12 g Protein, 2 g Fat)

TOTAL: 0 g Carbs, 12 g Protein, 2 g Fat

Takeaways: Lettuce is a great way to start a meal. Salad is so customizable that it can truly fit whatever cravings you may have. To mix things up, try different types of lettuce. If you get in a rut with salads, you're going to be turned off by them entirely. Experiment with different types of protein: chicken, steak, turkey. It's also easy to make your own dressing, so stay away from store-bought and save some money. I use a little extra-virgin olive oil, add a tablespoon of vinegar (balsamic, red wine, and white all work great), and then finish with freshly squeezed lemon juice, salt, and pepper. You can mix some in a bottle to keep in the refrigerator, or just mix directly on your salad. On top of being costly, those store-bought salad dressings are often loaded with sugar and additives and bad oils. Making your own helps you avoid the unnecessary calories and ingredients.

For dinner, it's a bison burger with air-fried "fries." Bison is a great, lean red meat. You may want to cook with ground beef or another red meat. Just make sure it's a lean cut and you don't overindulge.

DAY 5

BREAKFAST

Coffee, black (0 g Carbs, 0 g Protein, 0 g Fat)

¼ cup steel-cut oats (28 g Carbs, 7 g Protein, 3 g Fat)

½ cup blueberries (11 g Carbs, 1 g Protein, 0 g Fat)

1 cup unsweetened almond milk (0 g Carbs, 1 g Protein, 2.5 g Fat)

1 scoop zero-carb protein powder, vanilla (0 g Carbs, 25 g Protein, .5 g Fat)

Vegetable: 2 cups air-fried kale chips

TOTAL: 39 g Carbs, 34 g Protein, 6 g Fat

LUNCH

Greek Wrap:

3 oz. grilled chicken breast (0 g Carbs, 18.75 g Protein, 3 g Fat)

100% whole-grain tortilla (24 g Carbs, 6 g Protein, 3.5 g Fat)

5 Kalamata olives (2 g Carbs, 0 g Protein, 4 g Fat)

1 tablespoon tahini (1 g Carbs, 1 g Protein, 4 g Fat)

¼ cup fat-free feta cheese (1 g Carbs, 7 g Protein, 0 g Fat)

1 romaine lettuce leaf, chopped (0 g Carbs, 0 g Protein, 0 g Fat)

Vegetable: 1½ cups roasted Brussels sprouts

TOTAL: 28 g Carbs, 32.75 g Protein, 14.5 g Fat

DINNER

3 oz. rotisserie chicken, breast (0 g Carbs, 24 g Protein, 3 g Fat)

1 cup fingerling potatoes (30 g Carbs, 4 g Protein, 0 g Fat)

5 baby artichokes, roasted with olive oil and lemon juice (10 g Carbs, 4 g Protein, 4 g Fat)

Vegetable: 2 cups roasted green beans

TOTAL: 40 g Carbs, 32 g Protein, 7 g Fat

FLOATER MEAL

1 oz. leftover rotisserie chicken, breast (0 g Carbs, 8 g Protein, 1 g Fat)

TOTAL: 0 g Carbs, 8 g Protein, 1 g Fat

Takeaways: This floater meal is meant for after dinner and just before bed. This is for one of those "I'm still hungry, let's go raid the refrigerator" kinds of nights. Also great for those of you that still have some leftover rotisserie chicken from dinner. Just cut up a few pieces of the breast and eat it plain. I've never been afraid of cooking too much lean chicken because I know I'll make use of the leftovers. Even if I'm just cooking for myself, I know a rotisserie chicken will not go to waste because it is so versatile. Whenever I cook one, I immediately take all the chicken off the bone and separate the white meat from the dark meat. If I don't take it off the bones right away, I'll be less likely to eat the leftovers. I don't know about you, but a half-eaten animal carcass isn't too appealing when it's been sitting in the refrigerator. As soon as I take it off the bone, I weigh the meat I need for my meal and put the rest in a food storage bag in the refrigerator. I use the extra for my floater meal, or as a salad topping or to mix in with my Brussels sprouts. Don't be afraid of leftovers!

DAY 6

BREAKFAST

Coffee, black (0 g Carbs, 0 g Protein, 0 g Fat)

Egg White Omelet:

1 cup egg whites, cooked (0 g Carbs, 20 g Protein, 0 g Fat)

1 medium bell pepper (7 g Carbs, 1 g Protein, 0 g Fat)

1 cup spinach (1 g Carbs, 1 g Protein, 0 g Fat)

½ tablespoon coconut oil (0 g Carbs, 0 g Protein, 7 g Fat)

1.5 oz. salsa (3 g Carbs, 1.5 g Protein, 0 g Fat)

2 slices 100% whole-grain bread, toasted (30 g Carbs, 8 g Protein, 1 g Fat)

Vegetable: 2 cups air-fried kale chips

TOTAL: 41 g Carbs, 31.5 g Protein, 8 g Fat

LUNCH

Ground Turkey Lettuce Wraps:

4 oz. lean ground turkey (0 g Carbs, 22 g Protein, 6 g Fat)

¼ cup cooked black rice (15 g Carbs, 1.25 g Protein, 9 g Fat)

85 grams Greek yogurt aioli (nonfat Greek yogurt, lemon juice, garlic, salt, pepper) (5 g Carbs, 10 g Protein, 0 g Fat)

Vegetable: Small side salad

TOTAL: 20 g Carbs, 33.25 g Protein, 15 g Fat

DINNER

¾ cup brown rice pasta (32.25 g Carbs, 3 g Protein, 1 g Fat)

4 oz. lean ground chicken (0 g Carbs, 22 g Protein, 9 g Fat)

½ cup marinara sauce (7 g Carbs, 1 g Protein, 2 g Fat)

Vegetable: 2 cups roasted asparagus

TOTAL: 39.25 g Carbs, 26 g Protein, 12 g Fat

FLOATER MEAL

Nothing.

TOTAL: 0 g Carbs, 0 g Protein, 0 g Fat

Takeaways: Okay, you're probably look at this and thinking, "Why did you skip your floater meal?" Because you don't always need it. The three main meals here are satisfying enough, and maybe your Saturday workout was less intense than my weekday trips to the gym. Don't forget, the idea is to lose weight. If I'm not hungry, I don't eat. The floater meal is there for you when you need it, but it's not a requirement for the Super Carb Diet. Instead, I want you to think of it as your safety net.

DAY 7

BREAKFAST

Coffee, black (0 g Carbs, 0 g Protein, 0 g Fat)

3 slices turkey bacon (0 g Carbs, 6 g Protein, 7.5 g Fat)

1 cup egg whites, cooked (0 g Carbs, 20 g Protein, 0 g Fat)

2 slices 100% whole-grain bread, toasted (30 g Carbs, 8 g Protein, 1 g Fat)

½ cup blueberries (11 g Carbs, 1 g Protein, 0 g Fat)

Vegetable: 2 cups kale, sauteed

TOTAL: 41 g Carbs, 35 g Protein, 8.5 g Fat

LUNCH

3 oz. snapper (0 g Carbs, 22 g Protein, 1 g Fat)

1 cup cooked wild rice (35 g Carbs, 7 g Protein, 1 g Fat)

2 oz. avocado (4 g Carbs, 2 g Protein, 8 g Fat)

Vegetable: 2 cups roasted asparagus

TOTAL: 39 g Carbs, 31 g Protein, 10 g Fat

DINNER

1 cup chicken noodle soup (40 g Carbs, 9 g Protein, 2 g Fat)

2 hard-boiled eggs (0 g Carbs, 12 g Protein, 10 g Fat)

Vegetable: Add extra vegetables for a heartier soup

TOTAL: 40 g Carbs, 21 g Protein, 12 g Fat

FLOATER MEAL

3 slices turkey bacon (0 g Carbs, 6 g Protein, 7.5 g Fat)

1 hard-boiled egg (0 g Carbs, 6 g Protein, 5 g Fat)

TOTAL: 0 g Carbs, 12 g Protein, 12.5 g Fat

Takeaways: Cooking is always easier on the weekends. Most of you will have a little extra time in the mornings to make a fancy breakfast and meal prep for your lunch and dinner. When you're grocery shopping throughout the week, plan your weekends accordingly. If there's a new recipe you want to try that you haven't tackled yet, or one that is more time consuming, save it for Saturday or Sunday when you know time restraints won't discourage you. Making something tough on a Monday is going to make you feel defeated if it doesn't turn out properly. If it happens on the weekend, you can laugh it off and try something else without work looming in your mind. This also means buying your vegetables at the right time. If you do all your shopping on Monday and you need something fresh for a Saturday or Sunday meal, you may have to plan an extra trip to the supermarket later in the week.

I don't know about you, but I don't look at any of those meals and think, "boring." It's a full week's worth of breakfasts, lunches, and dinners that fall within the Super Carb equation. They aren't restrictive or dense. You should walk away from every one of those meals feeling satisfied and full. You can manage your plates exactly like I did, or you can customize to your own tastes. Don't like fish? That's fine. There are plenty of other protein options for you. Not a fan of brown rice? No problem. The possibilities are endless. I don't want you to feel like you can't eat. Yes, we are being strict, but that doesn't mean you are without options. You have three full meals, plus a floater meal that is going to ensure you don't go hungry. Again, don't feel the need to eat your floater meal every day if you aren't hungry for it. On days when you are away from the gym, you won't need the same amount of food as the days when you are pushing your limits on the rowing machine.

Keeping a food journal is a fantastic way to keep track of meals you like, and foods you don't. The numbers are going to keep you accountable on the Super Carb Diet, so you don't have to keep a diary of everything you eat, but it does help. Seeing all the things you eat written in front of your face is going to open your eyes in so many ways. One of the things I hear from friends who have tried my plan is that they had no idea they were eating so poorly before. A food journal is going to be an extension of that feeling. Once you see exactly what is going into your system, you won't believe how you spent so many years with those eating habits.

One other great benefit to keeping a food journal I haven't touched on yet. I'm talking about a second round of the Super Carb Diet. Have you ever done a cleanse or a program where you found great results, but afterward you fell off the wagon and started eating poorly again? Soon you've gained all the weight back and you're back where you started, The Super Carb Diet is a ninety-day plan. It's going to change your eating habits and open your eyes, all the while changing your body. After those ninety days are complete, it's up to you. But life happens. You have babies that change your body, you stress-eat after losing a job, you indulge on a vacation that throws you entirely off track or, like me, you have a heart attack. Those ninety worksheets you printed out at the beginning of this diet are going to be filled with numbers and foods. If you keep those worksheets in a journal during your ninety days on the Super Carb Diet, you can grab them during your second round to see exactly what you did the first time around. You'll know where you ran into trouble, or remember some recipes you particularly liked. That food journal is going to be your blueprint for taking the weight off again. Hopefully you won't need it. I truly want that to be the case. But like I said, life happens. The food journal is going to be another tool in your toolbox to get back on track for when your life gets in the way. None of this is easy, but if you don't stay diligent when life happens, you will spiral out of control. You must be willing to get back on the horse and try again when you fall off. If you have kept a food journal, it's going to be just a little bit easier to get back on that horse than if you need to start fresh without it. So, plan ahead. Be prepared. Don't allow yourself to spiral too far out of control.

17.

FAQs

You have all the tools you need to be successful. I'm giving you numbers to follow and rules to adhere to to help you on your Super Carb way. It's a lot of information. I get that. But remember, I want you to be successful. That's what drives me. I want to make sure you comprehend every little piece of the Super Carb Diet. I need you to be clear on everything, so you can get results and share your knowledge with others. To make sure you're all getting the bodies you always dreamed of, I've included this chapter with some frequently asked questions regarding the plan, as well as questions I get asked all the time. I love when you all come up to me on the street and want to know how to lose the last five pounds, or tap me on the shoulder on the subway to see what I think of new diet trends. Usually, if a health or fitness question is floating around in your head, it's floating around in the heads of a million other people. I gathered up as many of those questions as I could think of to include them here. This doesn't mean I want you all to stop coming up to me to chat, but maybe now we can chat about something other than health.

QUESTION: *I thought you're healthy. How did you have a heart attack?*

ANSWER: This has been the million-dollar question ever since I suffered a heart attack in February 2017. The truth is, even healthy people get heart attacks. It's an unfortunate truth. You can be the healthiest person on the planet, but there are still some unknown factors when it comes to heart attacks. What we do know is that there is genetic predisposition— meaning, you could carry a gene that makes you high-risk for a heart attack. My mother and grandfather both died of one, so it was something I was aware of, but many people are not. Nowadays, doctors can test for your genetic predis- position so you can be aware of your risk. Like I said before, it's also important to have these conversations with your living relatives while you can. I know everyone doesn't always have the best relationship with their parents or grandparents, but getting the information you need regarding their health history is important. It's also vital that you share that infor- mation with your primary care physician. Most doctors will ask when you go in for a physical. Be sure to let them know your family history so they can monitor what is needed. And for all the skeptics out there, know that you can work out and eat right, but still be at risk of a heart attack. What I want people to understand from my story is that practicing a healthy lifestyle will reduce your chances of heart disease AND give you a greater chance at full recovery if you do have heart issues. If you don't take care of yourself, you might not come out of that heart attack alive, let alone recover from it. Let's stack the deck in our favor as much as possible.

QUESTION: *Is it common for women to suffer from heart attacks or is it mostly men?*

ANSWER: YES! I think because movies and television always show men getting heart attacks that people tend to think women are immune. It's everyone. Male and female. In fact, heart disease is the leading cause of death for women in the United States. In 2013, 289,758 women died of heart disease, or about 1 in every 4 female deaths. And according to the American Heart Association, a heart attack strikes someone, male or female, about every 43 seconds.[1]

QUESTION: *I've always been told I should eat more in the morning than at night. Do you agree?*

ANSWER: It doesn't matter what time of day you're eating, just as long as it's balanced. On the Super Carb Diet, your meals will be mapped out for you based on your numbers. I doubt many of you will be eating your dinner AND your floater meal immediately before bed, but if you do, the numbers will keep you in check. When crafting this plan, I found that the balanced meals kept me satisfied throughout the day. If I ate a balanced plate for dinner, I wasn't as hungry when I went to bed at night. So often these diets will restrict certain meals. They'll tell you to have a light dinner or skip breakfast. That causes an imbalance, which inevitably hurts you at night. When the meals are balanced and spread out evenly throughout the day, you won't be starving at night or at four o'clock in the afternoon.

QUESTION: *I'm gluten-free; can I do the Super Carb Diet?*

ANSWER: YES! First, I want to stress that if you THINK you have a gluten allergy, you need to go to an allergist to get confirmation. Get checked and find out if it's for real. If it is, fine. Just because you are gluten-free does not mean you can't eat carbs. Fruit is gluten-free, but we know that there are also quite a bit of carbs in fruit. You can also have things like rice and quinoa, which are certainly not carb-free, but they are gluten-free. Don't let a gluten allergy dissuade you from the Super Carb Diet, because there are TONS of food options that remain.

QUESTION: *I'm vegan; can I do the Super Carb Diet?*

ANSWER: Yes. I was vegan for a long time, and I see lots of benefits in the lifestyle, particularly as it relates to heart health. On the Super Carb Diet, I want you using your body weight to calculate the amount of protein per meal. The protein source you eat is up to you. However, a lot of the protein options for vegans are also very high in carbs. If you're eating a protein like quinoa, you are getting some protein, but it's incredibly high in carbs. To reach both the balance in the numbers, you would need to have something like a pea protein supplement. It's doable. To make it easier,

I've included some vegetarian recipes in the back of this book.

QUESTION: *I don't have time to work out. Should I still try the Super Carb Diet?*

ANSWER: First of all, you should be able to find thirty minutes to work out three to five times a week. If you absolutely cannot do that, then you need to be even more strict with your carb, protein, and fat numbers. Carbs are fuel, but you won't need AS MUCH fuel if you aren't physically active. If that's the case, you need to lower your numbers to find what works for you to lose weight. Remember, I gave you a cap for your meals. Falling under those numbers is okay, particularly if you aren't actively working out. I prefer that you go to the gym, but we all go through times in our life when it isn't possible. If that happens during your ninety days, just cut back on your numbers.

QUESTION: *I'm injured, can I still work out?*

ANSWER: Of course. Do what you can. First, ask your doctor what you should and shouldn't do. If you are approved to go to the gym but worried about injuring yourself further, adjust. Tailor the workouts to fit your needs. After my heart attack, I could only do yoga, and my yoga skills were limited. So I adjusted. Eventually I could do more and more movements and exercises, but it was important to pace myself as my body healed. Be patient. An injury may set you back, but if you push too hard while injured, you'll suffer an even longer setback.

QUESTION: *Isn't a high-fat diet good for you?*

ANSWER: No. I've done the high-fat diets. You know, the ones where you can have unlimited bacon, but no bread. They tell you that you can eat all the red meat you want. No. That's not balanced. And it's also not realistic for a sustainable future. You may lose some quick weight and think it's working perfectly, but eventually, you're going to have carbs again. As soon as you do, the weight will start to come back quicker than ever. Don't try to trick your body into thinking a fat is a carb. It's not. A carb is a carb, and "carb" is not a dirty word.

QUESTION: *But I thought carbs are bad. . . .*

ANSWER: This isn't a question, but I hear it all the time. And NO! Carbs are not bad. They are fuel for our body. There's good carbs, and there's carbage. Stay away from the carbage and you'll be doing great.

QUESTION: *Can I juice my meals?*

ANSWER: Yes. And no. Make sure the juice is worth the squeeze. Pick a few meals a week that you want to juice. You can find recipes you like that incorporate the protein you need (using one of those protein powders we talked about), alongside the veggies, fruits, and nut butters to make it taste good. As always, be mindful of what you are putting in. Count every item you're liquefying. Some of those fruits are very high in carbs, so know that you need to limit them. I also don't want you buying your juices at juice bars. Those places will be a bit more lenient when it comes to measurements. Furthermore, they typically add extra fruit or nuts to make the juices taste good. The only way to be sure of what you're eating is if you make it yourself.

QUESTION: *When can I have a cheat meal?*

ANSWER: There are no cheat meals on the Super Carb Diet. You are getting well-rounded plates of food for breakfast, lunch, and dinner. Plus, I'm giving you that floater meal for when you need more sustenance. This diet plan is hard. You need to know that going in. In the end, it's worth it. You will be amazed at the changes your body makes. You'll even be amazed at the changes in your mental health and energy levels. These changes come at a price, and that price is giving up those crazy high-calorie meals that people refer to as cheat meals. That doesn't mean you can't have a slice of birthday cake ever again. This plan is for ninety days. I want you to give it everything you've got for those ninety days. After that, I'm confident you'll have the strength and know-how to balance your diet properly. A piece of cake will just be a piece of cake, and not a gateway into binge eating. This diet is going to show you how you were eating before so you know how to properly eat going forward. This isn't a diet plan for the rest of your life, but it will give you the tools you need to, hopefully, never need to diet again for the rest of your life. It's an investment in your future.

QUESTION: *I'm not in my twenties anymore; is the Super Carb Diet for me?*

ANSWER: YES. I'm fifty-one. FIFTY-ONE! If I can do it, so can you. The Super Carb Diet is for people of all ages. The numbers are customized to your specific body weight, and the food/menus are customizable based on your tastes/preferences. Anyone can do this plan, and everyone can be successful.

QUESTION: *Does is matter if I work out in the morning or at night?*

ANSWER: No. You can work out anytime you can fit it into your schedule. I prefer my workout in the morning because I get it out of the way and can enjoy the rest of my day without it lingering in the back of my mind. If you only have time after work or at nighttime, go for it. What I don't want you to do is put it off until it's too late. You know what I'm talking about. You say you're going to work out at night or after work, but then seven o'clock rolls around, you slowly put on your gym clothes while watching an episode of *Rachael Ray* that you DVR'ed with me as the co-host. Soon, it's eight o'clock and you haven't filled your water bottle. The clock strikes 8:45 and you decide it's best to just skip your workout for the day and go to bed early. We've all done it. That's why I want you to do the workout whenever you can, but try to schedule it every day accordingly. Put it in your calendar if that helps you remember. If you say you're going to work out at eight o'clock, then make sure you are walking in the gym doors at eight o'clock.

QUESTION: *When should I eat my floater meal?*

ANSWER: Whenever you want! I tend to have mine at night-time before bed because that's when I'm most hungry. Other times, I will have a zero-carb protein shake after an aggressive workout and count that as my floater meal. It's great for muscle recovery, so if my breakfast, lunch, or dinner doesn't fall after my workout, I'll have my floater meal as I'm leaving the gym. Whatever time you decide to eat it, just make sure you are only having protein and fat. It's NOT a full meal for you to load up on carbs.

QUESTION: *I'm on a budget, so what supplements do I absolutely need to take?*

ANSWER: A multivitamin. The other supplements I recommend in the micronutrient chapter are great, but if you absolutely cannot afford to buy all of them, stick with a good multivitamin. Make sure it contains 100 percent servings of the major vitamins, and make sure to take it every single day, preferably at the same time each day. If you have it at the same time each day, you'll get in the habit of taking it and you won't forget. If you can buy one other, I recommend magnesium. Take it at night and it will help you sleep soundly, and keep your digestive system working great.

Finally, next time you see your doctor for your yearly physical (you're all going for your yearly physical, right?), ask for supplement recommendations based on your health profile. Doctors will know better than anyone if you are lacking a nutrient. All our bodies are different, so you may find that you are missing something important for a variety of reasons.

QUESTION: *Some of the recipes are out of my carb, protein, or fat ranges per meal. Can I still have them?*

ANSWER: The recipes were created by me with my size in mind. I know not all of you weigh 185 pounds, so you'll have to adjust accordingly. As you're cooking, find ways to cut back if you need to by substituting ingredients or using less than the recipe calls for. If you need to add a few more grams of carbs, protein, or fat, increase the meat or veggies in the recipe. No one ever got fat eating leafy greens, so add them anywhere you can.

QUESTION: *My kids need to lose weight, what can I do?*
ANSWER: I always tell parents to start by making their kids lunches. It makes all the difference. Even though many schools around the country have moved toward a well-balanced plate, they still aren't perfect. Far from it. The only way to ensure that your kids are eating healthy at school is to pack lunch for them. Of course, you can't always be sure what your kids do with it once they're in school, but at least you have a start. Follow through by making well-rounded dinners and encouraging some form of exercise. Just get them moving. I know not all kids are into sports, but you must find something for them to do that will get them active. If your kids are gamers, buy them a game that will get them off their butts and moving while they play. (VR games are very interactive nowadays, and Nintendo has always made great games that encourage a lot of movement.) If your kid is into art and design, find a theater for him or her to join. Acting and stage management require a lot of movement. Do whatever you need to do to get kids moving and keep them active.

QUESTION: *How do I lose the last five pounds?*
ANSWER: I get this ALL the time. The infamous "last five pounds." People lose lots of weight, but can't seem to get rid of the last five to ten stubborn pounds that won't go away. For most of us, it's all in the stomach area, but maybe your stub-

born area is your arms or thighs. The truth is, you can run and lift weights like crazy, but those last few pounds are only going to come off in the kitchen. And in the kitchen, you need to make sure you are staying out of a rut. Switch up the foods you are eating, while remaining strict with your numbers, and try cutting back where you can. I don't mean you should starve yourself, but your body is smart. If you have been following a routine for a while, your body is going to stabilize and you'll find the pounds aren't coming off as easy as they once were. You need to surprise your body and be just a tad more intense when it comes to your diet. Just make sure you're doing it for the right reasons. Vanity is a great reason to get motivated, and it's often the only reason people start a diet. The goal, however, should always be health and wellness. I've found that some people are never happy with the way they look, so it may not be those last five pounds that are keeping you from being happy. All bodies are different. That's why some people have those beautiful round butts and tiny arms. Other people have flat butts and naturally muscular arms. Genetics play a huge role in how are bodies are formed, so there are going to be things that a diet cannot change. Those are the beautiful imperfections to embrace. If you are never fully satisfied with your body, find out what the deeper meaning is. And if there is no deeper meaning, and you just simply want to get those abs you've always dreamed of, then you need to work a little bit harder.

QUESTION: *How do I get a six-pack?*

ANSWER: Grocery stores usually put six-packs in the aisle with the wine and liquor. Like I said in the last question, to get the *abs* you always dreamed of, you will need to work just a little bit harder than usual. Six-pack abs are born in the kitchen, and they come at a price. It's attainable, for sure, but you must be strict. That means following the plan with no cheats and working out consistently. You may find that your body plateaus, in which case you will have to cut your calories and sugar intake even more to achieve those desirable abs. I know abs are what everyone wants, particularly in the summertime, but it takes a lot of work to get there. Most of the time when you see an Instagram model showing off their six-pack, they've been working on it for months or years. It doesn't happen overnight.

I always laugh when people tell me in April that they are getting ready to work on their summer body. The summer body needs to be worked on in the winter, not the spring. If you don't start until April, you won't even begin seeing those abs until the Halloween candy hits the store shelves. And we all know that Halloween candy means the Thanksgiving turkey is right around the corner, followed by the Christmas cookies and the New Year's champagne. The holidays are tough on our bodies, so you wind up never truly getting the summer bodies you want. So instead of looking for that summer six-pack in April, start early and keep at it. If you have the strength to avoid the holiday gluttony altogether, I encourage you to do so. It will help you get a summer body like never before. Once you have the summer body you always dreamed of, you'll be more encouraged to hold on to it for as many summers as you can.

QUESTION: *I've been doing the Super Carb Diet for a while, and I haven't lost any weight. What am I doing wrong?*

ANSWER: You may need to cut back on your numbers. The plate equation we figured out earlier is your cap. Those are the numbers I don't want you going over. If you are finding that you aren't losing weight, scale back your numbers a little bit more and see if you are getting results. Make sure you are counting your portions properly, and most importantly, reading the serving sizes on the foods you are eating. You may be eating way more than you think if you are reading that serving size wrong. If you are using one of those phone apps to keep track of your food, double-check the nutrition profiles each time you enter a food. I've found that many of those apps are user-generated, meaning people can enter nutrition facts and save to the system. For example, someone in Ohio may have calculated a chicken breast at 10 grams of carbs. When you search for chicken breast, it comes up and you choose it for yours. Their chicken breast may not have been the same as yours. Those apps are great for convenience, but you just need to double-check that you are not clicking and saving without looking twice. Get out your food scale. Measure. Be diligent. The weight will come off if you are doing those things.

QUESTION: *The contestants on* The Biggest Loser *lose weight so quickly. How is that possible?*

ANSWER: I get this all the time! People think that they should be able to lose weight as quickly as the contestants on *The Biggest Loser*. It's not realistic. Contestants are working on their weight loss twenty-four hours a day when they come on the show. It becomes their full-time job. They have the very best trainers, nutritionists, and doctors at their disposal. If you are expecting to lose weight as rapidly as they are, you're setting yourself up for failure.

In my book *Jumpstart to Skinny*, I said you could lose up to 21 pounds in 21 days. That diet plan was strict and formulated for just twenty-one days. On the Super Carb Diet, you have ninety days. It's still very strict, but the focus is on the marathon, not the sprint. Don't expect yourself to be down a pound each day when you weigh yourself. That's why I have you measuring your waist in addition to weighing yourself. On some days, you'll see the weight coming down on that scale number, and other days you'll notice the inches coming off the waistline. It's vital that you notice the results; this time I want you to notice them from more than just the scale.

QUESTION: *Isn't it better to eat a bunch of small meals instead of three big ones?*

ANSWER: In all my experience, I've found that when people are told they can eat a bunch of small meals, they aren't aware of how much food they are eating. Everything is spread out over such a long period that people lose track of what they've already had throughout the day. Keeping the bulk of your calories to three square meals will give you a better sense of the calories you are ingesting. It will also ensure that you are filling up during those three main meals so you don't have to keep snacking throughout the day. We don't want snacking.

QUESTION: *I have bad knees; can I still exercise?*

ANSWER: Talk to your doctor first. Always. If your doctor approves you for exercise, proceed with caution. If you are approved but still healing, you need to find exercises that work for you. If you have bad knees, I recommend staying away from running. I spent a lot of years running, and it was not great on my joints. Most days you'll find me at a CrossFit gym. I like CrossFit because the moves are always varied, the workouts are short, and I can scale accordingly. Most CrossFit gyms have great coaches that are certified and there to help you get through the workouts. Find a gym where people are there to help you. A good coach can let you know ways to scale back the workout depending on your injury or skill level.

QUESTION: *Isn't CrossFit bad for you?*

ANSWER: No. CrossFit sometimes get a bad rap for being some injury mecca. That's not true. You can injure yourself doing just about anything if you aren't careful. Which is why you need to be careful when/if you start CrossFitting. Find a box that has knowledgeable coaches. Compete with yourself, not with the people around you. People typically get injured doing CrossFit because they are trying to keep pace with the people around them. There's always going to be people with different athletic abilities than you. Instead of trying to keep up with them, adjust to fit your own needs. With ANY workout, be smart and careful.

QUESTION: *What's better for weight loss, cardio or weights?*

ANSWER: Both! When you reach your forties, your muscles start to deteriorate, so lifting weights is increasingly important as you age. Cardio is always great for burning calories; just be sure you aren't putting too much pressure on your joints. A lot of high-intensity cardio classes are popping up around the country, and I get worried. I worry because they are asking people to do intense sprinting at high inclines for short periods of time, which isn't great for the joints. Listen to your body.

QUESTION: *I've been working out for a while, but I still feel so out of shape. What can I do?*

ANSWER: Are you smoking? Don't smoke! I beg you, do not smoke. I know I didn't list it in any of the rules, but it's important. I'm telling you now. Stop smoking. If you do smoke, take these ninety days to make a conscious effort to quit. I find that's one of the main reasons people have trouble reaching their fitness goals. It's not good for your lungs or overall health, and it will hold you back when it comes to fitness. You also need to take a step back and analyze your fitness routine. Are you pushing yourself or are you doing what's comfortable and familiar? Not pushing yourself may be holding you back. Otherwise, just be patient. Working out is hard, especially when you are trying to eat healthy and take care of all the other things you have going on in your life. Give yourself some slack and some time. It will all come together if you stay focused and do the work.

With fitness, you need to make your goals small. Let's take pull-ups as an example. If you cannot do a pull-up, perhaps that's your goal. Most people will look at pull-ups and say, "I want to be able to do ten pull-ups." You may be at the gym for months and months without being able to complete one pull-up. If you set your goal too high, you will let yourself down and be more likely to give up entirely. You know the feeling of, "I can't do any, so why even try?" Instead, break it down even further. Make your goal simply to get up on the pull-up bar every day. Nothing more, nothing less. Once you have that down, try using a band for assistance. Every day just get up on that bar and do that much. Do it consistently until it is easy. Then drop to a band with less resistance. Do that every day until it is easy. You'll be getting stronger and eventually, try doing a single pull-up with no band. Try doing one a day, and build your way up to ten. It's frustrating that it takes so long, but it will work to your benefit. Achieving each tiny goal will give you a sense of accomplishment to keep going. You will see progress, and that progress will encourage you to keep moving forward.

QUESTION: *What should I look for in a trainer?*

ANSWER: If you are hiring a trainer, remember that trainers are working for you. Don't just throw your money at anyone. That means you can interview them and ask as many questions as you need to before hiring them. If they have a problem with that, move on to someone who doesn't.

The first thing I recommend asking them is what training certifications they have. I always see printed signs for personal trainers posted on telephone poles and subways. Occasionally, it will just be some muscly guy or girl looking to make a few extra bucks on the side without doing any schooling.

You will likely have to spend lots of money on personal training, so make sure you are getting a trainer that's worth it. You should also ask if they are CPR certified. It's great to know you have someone around who could save your life if you need it, AND it shows that they care about their work.

Once you sign up, be clear with what your goals are. Tell the trainer if you want to lose weight or just put on muscle. They can program the workouts accordingly. These criteria can be applied to finding a gym, too. If you are signing up for any sort of group fitness classes, make sure coaches are athletes who are able to live up to these requirements.

QUESTION: *What's the healthiest drink?*
ANSWER: Water. But if you're referring to alcohol, tequila and vodka are the best. Mix with soda water or drink straight on the rocks for the lowest calories. No sugary mixers.

QUESTION: *How much water should I drink in a day?*
ANSWER: At least five glasses per day. I recommend having a large glass before every meal, plus one as soon as you wake up. If it helps you, have a glass by the bed so you can drink it first thing in the morning. Also, be sure to stay hydrated when you're exercising. All that sweating is going to cause dehydration unless you get enough water. If you're always running late to the gym, fill up a water bottle at night and put it in the refrigerator before bed so you can just grab it and go before you work out the next day. I'm also a big fan of coconut water during exercise.

QUESTION: *What should I do after the ninety days are over?*

ANSWER: I made the Super Carb Diet ninety days because I want you to change your habits as you make changes to your body. If you follow the program, you will be thrilled with your results at the end of that time. You will also have the knowledge and power to keep going. Some people will continue, following it exactly as they did within the ninety days. You may need that structure to reach your goals. Other people will lose the structure but still find they are eating just about the same, without constantly measuring and adding. After the ninety days, you will know the amount of carbs, protein, and fat in the chicken breast you are preparing or the ground turkey you are buying. The structure may be gone, but the principles remain.

PART II
THE
TOOLS

FITNESS

You made it! You got through all the eating rules, the sleeping, and the math. But wait, there's more! I couldn't let you get off that easy. I need you to dust off that gym membership card, because fitness is important on the Super Carb Diet. If the food is the main dish of the Super Carb Diet, your exercise routine is the dessert. Or maybe it's the appetizer. Either way, your time at the gym is going to supplement everything you do in the kitchen. Those Thor biceps, Magic Mike abs, JLo booties, and beautiful Beyoncé/Bob Harper thighs are built in the gym. The food will help you reach your weight goals, while the exercise will help you define your body. Most of you know me from my workouts on *The*

Biggest Loser, so I want to make sure you have the info you need to be as successful in the gym as you are in the kitchen. After all, carbs and exercise go hand in hand. Don't want to take my word for it? the *New York Times* interviewed Oliver Neubauer, a senior research fellow at Queensland University of Technology in Australia, after a study he completed along with Jonathan M. Peake was published in the *Journal of Applied Physiology* regarding exercise and immunity. Mr. Neubauer states, "Ingesting carbohydrates during vigorous exercise may help, because carbohydrates maintain blood sugar levels. Having stable blood sugar levels reduces the body's stress response, which in turn, moderates any undesirable mobilization of immune cells."[1] He goes on to state, "Consuming carbohydrates in the first few hours immediately after strenuous exercise also helps to restore immune function." I don't recommend eating a bowl of pasta WHILE you're working out, but I do agree that carbohydrates are vital for active people. And guess what? You need to be active on the Super Carb Diet.

Before I get into my workouts, I need to talk about one rule I have when it comes to fitness: **Never enter a gym that doesn't have an automated external defibrillator (AED).** Well, you can enter one, but make sure you ask as soon as you enter if they have an AED machine and where it's located. I know that sounds dramatic, but I say it because I want ALL gyms to start carrying these machines, and it won't happen unless members start demanding them. Some states require gyms to have AEDs in their facilities, but others don't. It saved my life and it could save yours, too. AEDs are commonly found in public places where people gather, and chances are your gym already has one. However, most of the time they are placed on a wall or in a corner somewhere, never to be seen again. I want you not only to know whether your gym has one, but where it is located. When I went into cardiac arrest at my CrossFit gym in New York, I was lucky that they had an AED and that the instructor immediately knew where it was. When your heart is failing, a few seconds can make the difference between life or death.

It's not just gyms. I want AEDs to be everywhere. I'm calling on gyms, churches, businesses, and every location in between to invest in one of these machines. A friend recently reached out and told me his father saw me on television talking about AEDs. Right away his father went online and ordered one for his manufacturing facility in Northeast Ohio. Hearing that made me SO happy. If every one of you reached out to the people you know that have businesses of their own, imagine the lives we could save!

AUTOMATED EXTERNAL DEFIBRILLATORS (AED)

Most people I talk to about AEDs worry that they wouldn't know what to do if they had to use one. Trust me, they could not be easier. If someone enters cardiac arrest and you see the person collapse, first call 911 to make sure professionals are on their way. Then, locate the AED, turn it on (for most models, you just need to pull the plastic cover and it will turn on automatically) and let the machine instruct you from there. A voice will guide you. You want to make sure that the patient's clothes are removed from the chest area and there are no flammable liquids or standing water nearby. The AEDs also include printouts with visual directions, so you can see what you're doing while the voice instructs you. Easy, yes? If you are at a gym, ideally the trainers, coaches, and staff will be trained to use the equipment, but they are designed to be easy enough for anyone to use.

Why is an AED important if you can just call 911? According to the American Red Cross, the average response time is eight to twelve minutes for first responders once 911 is called.[2] That's on average, but it could certainly take longer. The chance of survival is reduced 10 percent for every minute that defibrillation is delayed. Every second is so crucial when someone enters cardiac arrest. Having an AED nearby can greatly improve your chance of survival before the paramedics arrive. This is the most important piece of equipment in the gym, and I am calling on every facility to have one available to their members. It's required by law in many states, but not all of them. If you are a gym owner and don't have one, hop online and order it. You can get them delivered next day and it can save lives. Furthermore, I urge all gym owners to talk to their staff and make sure they know where the AED is located and how to operate one. This must become part of the job training.

While we're talking training, I want to discuss CPR training. According to the *Journal of Emergency Medical Services,* for every minute that someone is unconscious and not breathing without CPR, they have a 10 percent less chance of survival.[3] You may have gotten CPR certified when you were a kid around the time you started babysitting, or perhaps you spent a summer lifeguarding and had to take a class. It would be GREAT if every single person were CPR certified. Unfortunately, that's not realistic. I do, however, want you to require your trainers and coaches to get their certification. Whether you're signing up for a CrossFit class or hiring a trainer on the side, you need to make sure your instructors have CPR training. Confirm that their certification is up to date. Oftentimes employees can provide proof of certification when they are hired, but they forget to renew after it expires. Techniques change, so certification typically only lasts for one or two years. If you are just getting renewed, organizations like the American Red Cross offer abbreviated courses for people that have been previously certified. When you're asking your trainers and coaches about their certification, be sure to ask when was the last time they took a class and if they are up to date.

Remember, gyms work for you. If you hire a trainer or sign up for a membership, you are paying them, so you need to make sure you are in good hands. Before you sign up, always ask if the facility has an AED and where it's located, and confirm that the staff is CPR certified. These simple questions can save your life, and if we start ensuring that our facilities have these base-level requirements, we can save the lives of those around us as well. If you saw me on TV after my heart attack, you saw me pledge to never set foot in a gym without an AED. I plan to stick to that. I made that proclamation on TV so that more people will join me in holding our workout facilities accountable. I no longer accept gyms who don't have these basic requirements, and you shouldn't, either.

My #BodyByBob classes are such a hit in New York and LA because anyone can do them, and everyone is challenged. Oftentimes fitness classes will cater toward elite athletes or people setting foot in the gym for the very first time. My classes welcome both. Not only is it a beautiful sight to see so many people of different fitness levels working together, but it also promotes healthy competition. So how do I cater my workouts to so many different types of gym rats? I use a mix of cardio and weights that can be easily scaled to your ability level. And the movements are constantly changing. This keeps the body alert, and you won't ever get bored. In all my years coaching and training clients I've noticed that sitting at a station for too long causes people to get complacent and slow. Slow is not going to burn the fat the way we want. I design my workouts with this in mind, ensuring that you're constantly moving. If you don't like a movement, don't worry because you're done with it quick. I kept all these workouts to around 30 minutes, so there's no excuse for you not to do them. I don't care who you are, you can make thirty minutes a day for three to five days a week happen. You may have to move some things around, but you can find the time. You wouldn't believe how often I hear people tell me they don't have time to work out. Usually people say this because they don't WANT to find the time to work out. It's easier to say they are busy than to rearrange a schedule.

If you follow me on social media, you know I'm a huge fan of CrossFit. I've been doing it for years because the workouts are constantly different, challenging, and quick. After my heart attack, I was asked if CrossFit is good for the heart. I believe that if you're doing any kind of workout, that's doing a lot more for your heart than sitting on the sofa. Like ANY workout, just be sure you have proper guidance and go at your own pace. Compete with yourself, not with the people around you. That doesn't mean I only do Cross-Fit. I'm always trying something new. Lately, I've been loving yoga and cycling classes. Just like I don't want you to get in a rut with your food, I don't want you to get in a rut with your workouts. Spice things up. Find a class or gym in your area and drag a friend along to try it. New scenery will keep you motivated. Sometimes all you need is a new facility to jump-start your fitness. I've provided some of my #BodyByBob workouts that you can do on your own in your gym of choice. Many of them you can even do at home. Wherever you decide to do it, I want you to work out three to five times a week. It's going to be hard at first. Many of you also will be adjusting to a completely new diet. If you've never worked out, this whole Super Carb Diet is going to be a lot of change, quick. If you want results right away, you'll need to push yourself at the gym right away. For those who want to make long-term changes, focus on the diet and slowly ease into the gym.

When it comes to working out, it's important to go at your own pace. I've started enjoying yoga lately because I've been doing it at my own speed. I used to hate it. I would get to a yoga class, look around at the people who do yoga every day, and try to do what they were doing. My competitive nature ruined it for me. Instead of accepting where I was at, I tried to push myself to be somewhere else entirely. After I had a heart attack, I was forced to go at my own pace. Yoga was one of the first workouts I was approved for, so I started taking classes every day. Now I spend the yoga class doing what I can and focusing on myself. I'm no longer looking around the room and trying to emulate the people around me. My goals have shifted to do the best that *I* can. I still look around the room from time to time to check out the beautiful people around me, but my competitive nature is no longer ruining the workout for me. I rest when I need to. I breathe. I adjust. And I encourage you all to do the same. You should never be embarrassed or feel bad about the level you're at. It's important to push yourself when you're try-ing to make changes to your body, but know that this is a marathon, not a sprint. You should feel challenged, but not overwhelmed. Rest when you need to. Breathe. Adjust.

I've included some of my favorite #BodyByBob workouts here

to get you started. These more than two weeks of scalable movements will burn an incredible number of calories. Some of them are the same program you would get if you stepped into one of my classes in LA or New York.

Some of the rehab workouts I did while I was healing are also here. I include them for those who need it. I was so lucky to have the time and resources to complete a cardiac rehabilitation program after my heart attack. Not everyone is so lucky. That's why I want to include some of the rehab workouts in this book. It's not just for heart attack survivors. You may be in perfect health now, but you never know when an injury will happen and you need a recovery-style workout. You'll also notice I give you my favorite hotel workout. This is the best thing to do when you're traveling and all you have is a tiny room and some workout shoes.

These exercises are ones I've done myself, plus the workouts I've used to train other people. I wish I could be there with you all, yelling and cheering you on, but you'll just have to use your imagination while you're working out without me. In those moments when you want to give up, picture me telling you to push a little harder. And remember, every time you dig a little deeper, your body is going to get a little closer to your goal.

You'll be sore. That's okay. Some of these workouts are TOUGH. I could've toned them down to make them easier for you, but I want to give you the tools I use to stay in the shape I'm in. None of this is supposed to be easy. It's not easy, but it's worth it. When your arms feel like Jell-O, put some ice on them. If your legs ache, use a foam roller to loosen them up before leaving the gym. Do whatever you need to do to push through and keep going because that's going to make all the difference when it comes to your body. You got this book, I'm assuming, to make a change in your life. Now's your chance to make that change. Work hard and don't give up. It's as simple as that.

GLOSSARY

AMRAP. This stands for "as many rounds as possible." When you see AMRAP listed in a workout, it means there is a set amount of time for that list of movements. The goal is to get as many rounds as you can of that list of movements within the given time. I challenge you to come back to these workouts. Mark your score down and try again after you've been in the gym for a while. Make sure you're improving.

Tabata. A training method that is 20 seconds of work, followed by 10 seconds of rest. Repeat that sequence for 8 rounds (a total of 4 minutes). It can be confusing, so let's break it down even further using air squats as an example. If I were doing a Tabata of air squats, it would look like this:

20 seconds air squats

10 seconds rest

20 seconds air squats

10 seconds rest

20 seconds air squats

10 seconds rest

20 seconds air squats

10 seconds rest

20 seconds air squats

10 seconds rest

20 seconds air squats

10 seconds rest

20 seconds air squats

10 seconds rest

20 seconds air squats

10 seconds rest

3-Tabata

TABATA: push-ups

Rest 1 minute

TABATA: air squats

Rest 1 minute

TABATA: sit-ups

SUPER TIP: There is no equipment required for this workout. It's 4 minutes of push-ups, 4 minutes of air squats, and 4 minutes of sit-ups. Be sure to rest a full minute between each Tabata. Air squats should be starting from a fully upright position and squatting down to below 90 degrees from your knees. For the sit-ups, do them on an ab mat or a yoga mat for maximum butt comfort.

Minute by Minute

1 minute jumping jacks

1 minute mountain climbers

1 minute inch worms

1 minute plank hold

1 min alternating lunges

Rest 1 minute

Repeat 4 times.

SUPER TIP: This is another workout that you can do without any equipment. If you have a yoga mat, I recommend using it for all the movements. It will be good to have some cushioning for your knees and elbows. For my advanced people, you can do the lunges with weight. For instance, if you have two dumbbells, you can hold one in each hand as you do your alternating lunges. However, these are supposed to be fast, so only use the weight if you can do the movement quickly. I want your heart rate to get up, so don't treat any of it as a warm-up.

Death by Jump Rope

Max jump rope for 30 seconds

Max sit-ups for 30 seconds

Max jump rope for 60 seconds

Max sit-ups for 60 seconds

Max jump rope for 90 seconds

Max sit-ups for 60 seconds

Max jump rope for 120 seconds (2 minutes)

Max sit-ups for 60 seconds

Repeat 1–2 times

SUPER TIP: I LOVE jumping rope. It's a fantastic way to get your heart rate up. For this workout, you'll notice I capped the sit-ups at 60 seconds. I want you moving fast when you're doing them. For my beginners, repeat the entire sequence one time through. For my advanced athletes, do it twice. And remember, use a yoga mat if you have one to protect your caboose during the sit-ups.

WORKOUT #4

Step Challenge

10 step-ups on and off a 12–20-inch box, depending on your ability

20 lunges off the top of the box

30 air squats

10 step-ups on and off the box

30 air squats

Rest 2 minutes

Repeat

SUPER TIP: For this workout, you'll need a 12–20-inch box. Most gyms have these now, but if you do not have one, replace the step-ups with 1 minute of jumping rope. For my beginners, simply step all the way on top of the box and then step down. Advanced athletes can do box jumps. These jumps are a faster movement, and it's important to be extra careful when performing this move. One small mistake and you can fall and hurt yourself. For the lunges, beginners can use no weights, and advanced athletes should use weights (dumbbells in each hand).

WORKOUT #5

Bicycle Intervals

Bike for distance for 1 minute

Rest 1 minute

Repeat 10 times

SUPER TIP: For this workout, you'll need an upright stationary bike. Bike as far as you can for 1 minute. Write down your distance. Rest for 1 whole minute. Bike another minute. Your goal is to hit the same distance or BETTER than you did in that first minute. You'll do this for 10 rounds (20 minutes total). For my advanced athletes, I'd like you to shoot for 15 or 20 rounds (30 or 40 minutes total). Always be sure to rest one full minute after bicycling for a minute. You also want to be sure to keep track of that first distance and try your best to hit that same distance or better each round. The goal here is endurance, so it should be TOUGH to go the same distance by round 10.

Kettlebell Hell

10 kettlebell swings

20 goblet squats

30 reverse lunges with kettlebell

1 minute of jump rope

Rest 1 minute

Repeat 3–5 times

SUPER TIP: Kettlebells are a great tool to have at your home gym. They are so versatile. For this workout, there are a few ways to customize based on your ability. For the swings, you can either swing to eye level or overhead, using the weight of your choice. When you get to the lunges, you can hold the kettlebell in the goblet squat position, or you can hold it on your side, depending on your ability. If you are a beginner, substitute jumping jacks for the jumping rope. I say 3–5 rounds because I want you to customize based on your time and ability. If you have extra time, do extra rounds. Furthermore, use a kettlebell that is going to challenge you but still allow you to move quickly. We want your heart rate elevated, so don't choose a weight that is going to slow you down.

WORKOUT #7

Thruster Duster

20 dumbbell thrusters

Hold squat 30 seconds (with weights on shoulder)

Stand and hold weights overhead for 30 seconds

Repeat 3–5 times

SUPER TIP: This workout won't take up a lot of space. You just need a pair of dumbbells. They should be a challenging weight, anywhere from 10 to 45 pounds, depending on your strength level. If you are looking to build muscle and want to use a heavier weight, be sure to do so under supervision. Thrusters are a very taxing movement. They work your legs, core, shoulders—the entire body. They are brutal. A bad form will hurt your back and cause you weeks of pain. Be careful! If these moves are new to you, scale back and do the moves you are comfortable with. For thrusters, you can start by going through the movement slowly to work your way up to a full rep. Use light weights until you are accustomed to the thruster.

For the squat holds, put the dumbbells on your shoulders. If you are a beginner, you can simply hold a squat for 30 seconds without any weight. When you are standing and holding the weights overhead for 30 seconds, be sure to lock out your elbows. Your arms should be straight, as should your spine. If you round your back and injure yourself, it will set you back weeks, so only use a weight you know you can work with for 3–5 rounds.

WORKOUT #8

Ball Slams

20 ball slams in 1 minute

Rest for the remainder of the minute

Repeat 5 times

30 ball slams in 1 minute

Rest for the remainder of the minute

Repeat 5 times

SUPER TIP: This is a 10-minute workout, and it sneaks up on you. Find a medicine ball at a doable weight and a small corner of the gym. You'll also need a stopwatch. You can use your phone app to keep the time, or have a friend time and count for you. For the slams, take the ball completely overhead and slam it to the ground. The goal is to catch it as it bounces up, then repeat the movement until you get to 20 in the first minute. Any remaining time you have in that minute is yours to rest. When minute 2 starts, pick up that ball again and do 20 more. You'll go through 5 rounds of 20 (5 minutes) and 5 rounds of 30 (5 minutes). This workout is a great "friend" workout. You can alternate and count for each other, making sure you're each accountable. I don't know about you guys, but I LOVE to work out with friends. You can motivate each other and it's helpful to have an extra set of eyes on you to ensure proper form.

WORKOUT #9

Core Blaster

AMRAP 20–30 minutes

10 push-ups

20 mountain climbers

10 air squats

20 sit-ups

Rest 1 minute

SUPER TIP: This AMRAP should be 20–30 minutes, depending on your skill level. My advanced athletes should be doing it for 30 minutes, especially because it's all body-weight movements. You'll notice that I have a 1-minute rest in each round. This is nonnegotiable. The first round you may find easy and be tempted to skip the rest time. Don't. By the end of the 20 (or 30) minutes, you will be tired. The rest is programmed to make sure your body can make it the entire time. I also want to make sure you all write down how many rounds you get when you are doing this workout. You can jot it in this book if you need to, just be sure to write the number somewhere. Then try the workout again after a few weeks to compare. You should be getting better, not worse. Keep yourself accountable. These workouts are ones that you can come back to. Keep a journal regarding how you do with each. Every time you do the same workout, you should be doing just a little bit better.

Tread Rehab

3-minute walking warmup on treadmill (speed 3.0–4.0 mph)

8 minutes at a 7° incline and an increased speed of .5 mph (3.5–4.5 mph)

2 minutes at a 10° incline and same speed (3.5–4.5 mph)

2-minute cool down at 0° incline at your starting speed (speed 3.0–4.0 mph)

Rest 2 minutes

Repeat

SUPER TIP: This is one of the rehabilitation workouts I did after my heart attack. I love the gym. After my cardiac arrest, my doctors wanted me to slowly ease back into my workout routine. They designed rehab workouts for me to build my stamina so that I could train the way I always had. This is one of those workouts. For me, it was what I considered rehabilitation, but it's a fantastic workout for beginners who haven't been to a gym before. It's a great way to start building your endurance before attempting a higher-intensity workout. Plus, the slower speeds will ensure you aren't putting too much pressure on your knees. I always caution runners to be careful on the treadmill at those crazy-high speeds because it can be very brutal on the joints, especially if you aren't a trained runner.

WORKOUT #11

Straight-up Cardiac Rehab

Pick any 3 pieces of cardio equipment in the gym (treadmill, bike, rower, elliptical, step mill, etc.) and spend 15 minutes on each machine.

SUPER TIP: I lied when I said we were finished with all the math. This workout DOES require a little bit of math, but it's for good reason. I did this 3 days a week to strengthen my heart after my heart attack. This requires a gym facility (or a home gym with at least 3 cardio machines). Pick 3 and spend 15 minutes on each one, keeping your heart rate around 60–70 percent of your max heart rate for 10 of the 15 minutes. To get your max heart rate: $220 - \text{your age} = \text{max heart rate}$. At age 51, that means my max heart rate is 169 ($220 - 51 = 169$).

The key is to start with 3 minutes of warming up and spend the last 2 minutes cooling down on EACH piece of cardio equipment. Let's say I picked a rower as my first piece of cardio equipment. I would get on the rower and spend 3 minutes warming up at a light/moderate speed. At the start of minute 3, I want to make sure my heart rate is 60–70 percent of that max heart rate I calculated earlier. Once I enter that zone, I would row at the same pace for 10 minutes. Then I would spend the last 2 minutes cooling down at a light/moderate pace. You'll do that same pattern for 2 other pieces of cardio equipment. Like I said, this one requires some math, but once you get the hang of it, it will seem easy to calculate. I love this workout because you can always change it up. If I get tired of the rower, I can skip it and do a treadmill, bike, and elliptical sequence. I've heard from so many people since my heart attack who have gone through similar situations, and they always ask what kind of workouts they can be doing to start working out again. This is my favorite because it becomes a game when I enter the gym and get to decide which equipment to use.

Weight Rehab

15 chest presses

15 shoulder presses

15 single-arm rows

15 single-arm tricep extensions

15 bicep curls (palms facing up)

15 chest flies

15 lateral arm raises

15 bent-over rows

15 single-arm overhead tricep extensions

15 hammer bicep curls (palms facing each other)

Repeat 3 times

SUPER TIP: These workouts are all about cardio rehab, and this one is targeting weight rehab. It's all about the fundamentals. When I was rehabilitating, I was required to do this workout with 10-pound weights. I thought it was going to be superlight, but it turned out to be challenging because there are so many movements. Anyone who has had rehab after a medical setback knows that your mind isn't quite on the same wavelength as your body. This is all about focusing on each exercise at a light weight. I used to be able to clean and jerk 225, so when my trainers had me doing this workout with 10-pound weights, it was a blow to my ego. I found out that it was incredibly beneficial for me to go back to basics and focus on form.

Advanced athletes can modify this workout and use heavy weights—I promise it will be a challenge to anyone. For this workout, keep track of the time it takes to do one full round. You will be doing a total of four, so I want you to make sure you are staying consistent with your times. I also want you to come back to this workout and see if you're able to do it faster or with heavier weights after you've been training for a few weeks. See how you progress.

The Best Exotic Hotel Workout

100 burpees for time

SUPER TIP: People are always asking for my favorite vacation workout. This is it. It is crazy challenging. You may need to build yourself up to 100. If that's the case, try doing 50 and see how you feel. You don't need any equipment, and you can do it anywhere, so there's no excuse not to break a sweat when you're spending a few days by the beach or in a tiny hotel room.

That's it. Thirteen workouts. That's over two weeks of fitness on the Super Carb Diet. They can be scaled to your ability, and all of them should be done with caution. If you are new to working out, then start small. Use lighter weights. Listen to your body. Talk to your doctor. One of the things I notice in clients who have never worked out before is that they tend to get discouraged when they can't do something. We are ALL at different levels. After my heart attack, I had to start at square one. I was doing beginner workouts for weeks. Once I got over myself and committed, I noticed I was getting stronger and stronger. I had to reconcile with the need to go slow and focus on my rehabilitation. I kept making progress, and I continue to make progress.

Don't get discouraged. You will have days that are tough, but there will also be days that you feel motivated to hit the gym. Some mornings you will wake up sore. That's all a part of it. Stretch. People always forget to stretch. You should stretch before your workout, and after your workout. It's annoying sometimes because it's extra time at the gym, but it will make a difference. Breathe. Take a yoga class. If you've never taken one before, you can usually try your first one for free. Use a foam roller to loosen your muscles. You can buy one online for less than ten dollars. It's a worthy investment. Get a massage. Or better yet, get some massage lotions and oils for home. Ask your significant other to massage your sore muscles so you can save some money. Celebrate the small victories. If you've never worked out before, be proud when you complete a workout. If you have been an athlete all your life, be proud that you took the time to make progress. Find ways to make fitness work for you and I promise you will get results.

RECIPES

I love to cook. When I'm in the kitchen, I can set my mind to a task and forget everything else I have going on. It's therapeutic. When I set out to create the Super Carb Diet, I did a lot of experimentation. I played with my numbers and, as a result, played with my recipes. Certain go-to's that I would make in the kitchen didn't work for me anymore, while new foods I had never worked with before suddenly became staples. After my heart attack, I cut back on meats drastically and had to learn new ways to cook leaner proteins and vegetables. The Super Carb Diet forced me to play in the kitchen.

Anytime you try a new diet, it's a great opportunity to try foods you have never tried before. Often I hear from clients that they are getting bored. Bored with their food choices. They eat the same foods for breakfast, lunch, and dinner to try to lose weight. We've all met or been that person before. You know, the one who has a shake for every meal and carries around rice cakes to snack on, every single day. People think being on a diet means they must eat boring food. That's wrong! You can change up food at every meal. If you're someone who *likes* to eat the same thing for every meal and would rather do that than cook each meal, feel free. For everyone else, don't get in a kitchen rut. You can have the most beautiful, flavorful food when you step outside your comfort zone.

I know what you're thinking: Cooking takes time, and we don't have a lot of it. We have sleeping, and carpools, and school, and work. There are so many other things we need to do throughout the day that cooking oftentimes gets lost in the shuffle. The Super Carb Diet is strict for a reason—to get you results! Because there's no easy way to lose weight. Unfortunately, we can't take a shortcut in the kitchen. Cooking must become part of your routine if you want to make changes. I've been thinking about how to motivate you in the kitchen. I know you all want to lose weight, but you want the kitchen shortcuts. I understand. I do, too. Unfortunately, you have to do some cooking on my plan without a lot of time-savers. There's no way around it. Instead of lying to you, I want to get you to start thinking of cooking in a different way.

Most of us watch TV. You may only have bought this book because you've seen me on television. We sit in front of our screens to relax with some of our favorite shows about doctors, good wives, housewives, fuller houses, houses of lies, and houses of cards. Just like you think about relaxing with your favorite shows, I want you to start thinking of relaxing via *cooking*. When you're in the kitchen, focus on the meal in front of you and let all of life's worries melt away for that short time. Begin to enjoy the recipes. Start to reprogram your mind so that cooking becomes a hobby instead of a chore. Make it the centerpiece of your date night, or instead of meeting friends at the movie theater, have everyone bring over an ingredient and cook together. Time in the kitchen is an investment in your future. The healthier you cook, the happier you'll be.

The recipes in this section are all ones that I love, my absolute favorites. They include the balanced foods and recipes I've discovered on my Super Carb journey. Do they include everything? Hell no. You won't see a lot of "dessert" foods here because this diet isn't designed for you to have dessert. Sure, there are things like muffins and macaroons that you can craft to fit into your Super Carb plate, but I don't want you to think that way. If you have one of those "healthy" desserts, it will come at the cost of the healthy foods you should be eating. Like the vegetables. That said, there are a couple of sweeter recipes you can try, but I don't want you to think of them as dessert. And don't let these specific recipes limit what you have available on your own. Go out and explore the supermarket. Find foods you've never had before, experiment with these recipes by adding ingredients you like and taking out the ones you don't. These recipes might not fit into your Super Carb plate perfectly because they are tailored to my numbers. You'll have to adjust. Eat less, or eat more, depending on *your* numbers. Think of these recipes as templates for you to get started. I want you to keep track of your numbers, but don't let that stop your creativity.

After you lose the weight, you'll have the body you always wanted, and it will need to be maintained. To maintain it, you'll need to eat healthy, and that means you'll need to keep cooking. Sure, there are lots of healthy restaurants out there, but if you cook at home, you'll know, with 100 percent certainty, what is in your food. Be mindful of your ingredients, but make these recipes your own. And when you do, and you make something you're proud of, share it with me on social media. I get a lot of snarky comments online when I post a photo of my food (#ImAChef), but oftentimes those same people that laugh at my chicken and Brussels sprout recipe will send me pictures of their own version of it. A variation you create may spark an idea for me, and I hope some of these recipes spark an idea for you. Please, take these recipes, mold them to your palate, and create dishes I've never seen before.

A lot of people ask me what my favorite kitchen tools are. If you're new to cooking, you'll need to stock up on the essentials. There are so many different appliances to choose from. Wading through all the great gadgets can be tough. I've made a list of some of my favorites. Are these necessities? No. These are the items I've found over the years to be most helpful to find success in the kitchen. I left off the most common items, the frying pan, measuring cups, and so forth. I'm assuming you already have those. We talked about the food scale, so I left that off as well. These are the rest of my favorite kitchen essentials to get you cooking:

1. **AIR FRYER.** This has become my new favorite kitchen toy. It's fantastic for getting crisp vegetables and low-fat meats. I'm a Southern boy, so I love the flavor of anything fried, but obviously the traditional fried method is no good for us. The air fryer gives you the taste of fried, without the side effects. When you're using one, just be sure to leave enough room and give a quick spray of oil to ensure the foods don't stick after cooking.

2. **SLOW COOKER.** If you're busy, and I know you are, a slow cooker will become your best friend. You can throw your ingredients in, leave for work, and come home to a delicious meal that is ready to eat. A slow cooker is great for stews and meat. On the Super Carb Diet you'll be eating a lot of lean meats, and a slow cooker is a fantastic way to get the most flavor out of those lean meats and ensure they don't dry up when you're cooking them. There's even "smart" cookers now that connect to your phone so you can always be in control of the cooking.

3. **SOUS-VIDE COOKER.** Okay, this one is fairly new to me, but I LOVE it. These cookers are popping up in more and more stores, and for good reason. A sous-vide machine is a contraption that plugs into your wall and goes into a large pot filled with water. You throw your food in a sealed plastic bag, immerse it in the pot of water, set your temperature, and let it cook. The reason I like the sous-vide method of cooking is that it allows the meat and vegetables you cook to retain moisture. Like the slow cooker, it's great for lean meats. No more dry chicken breasts. Plus, you get all the juiciness of the food without adding all the oil you would when cooking it in a pan.

4. **SPIRALIZER.** I'm not going to lie and tell you zucchini noodles are as good as traditional pasta noodles. They aren't. That doesn't mean they are bad, just different. A spiralizer will allow you to make those fresh zucchini noodles for pasta-esque meals. Lots of grocery stores are selling veggie noodles prepackaged, which is great,

but they are always way more expensive than just buying the vegetable and spiraling them yourself. If you have the room in your kitchen and the time to spiral, I recommend picking up one of these. You can also use it for carrots, potatoes, and more.

5. **BLENDER/MIXER.** Some days a liquid lunch is all I have time for. I throw a couple scoops of protein powder, some nut butter, fruit, and almond milk into my blender and I have a great meal that's balanced and delicious. The NutriBullet Magic Bullet is great because you can blend and easily detach the blending cup to take on the go without having to transfer the smoothie to another cup. It also is strong enough to blend fruits and vegetables that have a tougher texture for making juices and smoothies.

5. **MEAL CONTAINERS (TUPPERWARE).** You're going to be doing a lot of cooking over the next ninety days, and you're busy. Buying food containers that you can reuse is going to save you so much time! You can do cooking at the beginning of the week and have meals ready for you each day instead of trying to figure out something new every day at lunchtime. I know I said variety is going to keep you from getting in a rut, but I also know a lot of you out there are creatures of habit. Meal prep has always been a secret weapon for athletes. I'm sure you've seen those fitness models you follow on Instagram who post pictures of their meal prep. You know, the ones with seven containers filled with grilled chicken breast and broccoli every Sunday. On the Super Carb Diet, you don't have to eat the same thing for every meal, and

I hope I've encouraged you to try new foods. However, I'm one of those creatures of habit. I can eat the same thing for every meal if I have to. Meal-prep containers will make it easy for you to whip up a balanced meal you like when you have the time to make enough to last you through the week, and then you will have your Super Carb plate packaged and ready to go.

These specialty kitchen gadgets are my favorites. Of course, you can get by with just a frying pan and some salt and pepper, but these gadgets will make the ninety days of food prep a little bit easier. Every little bit helps, right? Now the only thing left to do is get cooking. The nutrition facts are PER SERVING, so please note that when you're cooking. If you're unsure, grab a piece of paper and a pen and do the math yourself. Foods tend to vary based on the brands you buy and the types you use, so ALWAYS calculate the numbers yourself so you can be sure you are crafting your plate properly. You'll also find some great options in my other books. There's a large selection of recipes in my book *The Skinny Rules* that are easily customizable for the Super Carb Diet, so be sure to check it out.

EGG WHITE TOWER SANDWICH

*MAKES 1 SERVING

1 TEASPOON COCONUT OIL

1 CUP EGG WHITES

SALT

PEPPER

2 SLICES 100% WHOLE-GRAIN BREAD

⅛ AVOCADO

½ CUP SALSA

Heat coconut oil in frying pan.

Beat egg whites with salt and pepper.

Once pan is hot and oil is melted, add egg whites to pan and cook to desired consistency.

Toast bread.

Once toasted, layer bread, avocado, and egg white equally in three layers.

Add salsa to top.

NUTRITION INFORMATION ■ 37 G CARBS ■ 34 G PROTEIN ■ 5 G FAT

LEAN GROUND TURKEY BURRITO

*MAKES 1 SERVING

1 TEASPOON COCONUT OIL

4 OZ. LEAN GROUND TURKEY

1 CUP BROCCOLI, FINELY CHOPPED

1 LOW-CARB TORTILLA

2 ROMAINE LETTUCE LEAVES (A HANDFUL OF CHOPPED LETTUCE WORKS GREAT, TOO)

½ CUP SALSA

Heat coconut oil in frying pan.

Once hot, add ground turkey and broccoli. Cook until meat is brown.

Add to tortilla with lettuce and salsa.

Enjoy!

NUTRITION INFORMATION ■ 26 G CARBS ■ 31 G PROTEIN ■ 14 G FAT

CHICKEN WITH SHAVED BRUSSELS SPROUTS

*MAKES 3 SERVINGS

2 TABLESPOONS OLIVE OIL

4 OZ. SKINLESS CHICKEN BREAST

2 CLOVES GARLIC, PEELED AND CHOPPED

10 OZ. SHAVED BRUSSELS SPROUTS

¼ SWEET ONION, PEELED AND CHOPPED

SALT

PEPPER

Heat 1 tablespoon olive oil in frying pan.

Cook chicken breast on medium heat. Remove from pan.

Add 1 tablespoon olive oil and chopped garlic to pan.

Once garlic is heated, add Brussels sprouts and onion.

Cook shaved brussels sprouts until they begin to brown and onion is translucent.

Cut chicken into small pieces and add to pan.

Add salt and pepper.

Mix and enjoy!

NUTRITION INFORMATION ▪ 11 G CARBS ▪ 11 G PROTEIN ▪ 12 G FAT

SUPER NOTES

I LOVE to add Canadian or turkey bacon to this recipe. Just cook 1–2 slices before cooking the chicken, and instead of using the olive oil, cook the chicken and vegetables in the leftover bacon grease. I prefer the bacon finely chopped.

VEGAN STUFFED PEPPER

*MAKES: 1 STUFFED PEPPER

½ CUP VEGGIE GROUND BEEF

⅔ CUP CAULIFLOWER RICE

½ CUP TOMATO SAUCE

1 TABLESPOON OLIVE OIL

1 LARGE BELL PEPPER

Heat veggie ground beef, cauliflower, and tomato sauce in olive oil in the frying pan.

Cut off stem of red pepper and remove seeds.

Fill pepper with mixture and bake at 375 degrees for 30 minutes.

NUTRITION INFORMATION ▪ 39 G CARBS ▪ 27 G PROTEIN ▪ 14 G FAT

SUPER NOTES

Veggie ground beef is great for vegetarians. I like to use bell peppers, but you can certainly substitute with your favorite pepper and adjust.

VEGAN SLOPPY JOE

½ CUP VEGGIE GROUND

¼ CUP TOMATO SAUCE

1 WHOLE-GRAIN BUN

1 TEASPOON OREGANO

SALT

PEPPER

Cook veggie ground over medium heat in frying pan with tomato sauce.

Season with oregano and desired amount of salt and pepper.

Once cooked, put mixture in bun and enjoy!

NUTRITION INFORMATION ■ 35 G CARBS ■ 27 G PROTEIN ■ 13.5 G FAT

SUPER NOTES

This tastes great with diced peppers or onions added if you have them left over from one of your other recipes. Be sure to have some napkins handy, because it gets messy!

BOB'S FAVE PROTEIN DRINK

SERVING SIZE: 8 OZ.

1 SCOOP VEGAN PROTEIN POWDER

½ FROZEN BANANA

1 TABLESPOON ALL-NATURAL NUT BUTTER

½ CUP UNSWEETENED ALMOND MILK

2 ICE CUBES

Throw everything in a blender and ta-da!

NUTRITION INFORMATION ■ 30 G CARBS ■ 24.5 G PROTEIN ■ 15 G FAT

GREEK YOGURT PARFAIT

*MAKES 1 SERVING

¾ CUP FRESH MIXED BERRIES

¼ TEASPOON CINNAMON

1 CUP NONFAT PLAIN GREEK YOGURT

1 TABLESPOON ALL-NATURAL PEANUT BUTTER

Mix fresh berries and cinnamon with Greek yogurt.

Top with 1 tablespoon of peanut butter.

Enjoy!

NUTRITION INFORMATION ▪ 37 G CARBS ▪ 17 G PROTEIN ▪ 8 G FAT

SUPER NOTES

Have you noticed how much I love my Greek yogurt? Jamie Lee Curtis and John Stamos should invite me to their next group meeting.

FISH TACOS

½ TEASPOON CAYENNE PEPPER

½ TEASPOON CUMIN

SALT

PEPPER

3 OZ. MAHI-MAHI

1 TEASPOON OLIVE OIL

1 LOW-CARB TORTILLA

¼ CUP SALSA

¼ JALAPEÑO, MINCED

¼ YELLOW ONION, PEELED AND CHOPPED

2 TABLESPOONS FRESH CILANTRO, CHOPPED

In mixing bowl, combine cayenne pepper, cumin, salt, and pepper.

Rub mixture over mahi-mahi.

Heat olive oil in a pan on medium heat and cook.

Once cooked, place in tortilla and add salsa, jalapeño, onion, and cilantro, to taste.

Enjoy!

NUTRITION INFORMATION ▪ **19 G CARBS** ▪ **21 G PROTEIN** ▪ **8 G FAT**

HAM AND EGG BREAKFAST BURRITO

*MAKES 1 SERVING

1 TEASPOON OLIVE OIL

¾ CUP EGG WHITES

SALT

PEPPER

1 LOW-CARB TORTILLA

1 OZ. NITRATE-FREE HAM

Heat olive oil in pan.

Cook egg whites to desired consistency with salt and pepper.

Remove egg from pan and heat tortilla.

Once hot, remove from pan and wrap ham and egg in low-carb tortilla.

Enjoy!

NUTRITION INFORMATION ▪ 15 G CARBS ▪ 31 G PROTEIN ▪ 9 G FAT

FROZEN GRANOLA CAKES

12 CUPCAKE LINERS

12 OZ. ORGANIC ROLLED OATS

32 OZ. NONFAT GREEK YOGURT

1 CUP MIXED FRESH BERRIES

Line cupcake or muffin pan with liners.

Fill bottom with oats.

Add Greek yogurt on top of oats.

Put berries on top of yogurt.

Freeze for 1–2 hours.

Enjoy frozen, or let them thaw for a short time if you prefer a softer texture.

NUTRITION INFORMATION ▪ 13 G CARBS ▪ 10 G PROTEIN ▪ 1 G FAT

SUPER NOTES

I love my nonfat Greek yogurt, and these are great for when I'm on the go. Some days I just don't have the time to mix my oats and fruit, so having them ready-to-go and in the freezer for when I'm heading out the door is a plus. You can also customize these with your favorite fruits or nuts, or a healthy cereal you like in place of the oats. They make great snacks for the kids.

CHICKEN MEATBALLS

*MAKES 4 SERVINGS

1 LB. LEAN GROUND CHICKEN

1 EGG, BEATEN

2 TABLESPOONS MILLED FLAXSEED

2 CLOVES GARLIC, PEELED AND MINCED

1 TEASPOON OREGANO

1 TEASPOON RED PEPPER FLAKES

1 TEASPOON SALT

1 TEASPOON PEPPER

1 TABLESPOON OLIVE OIL

WATER

Preheat oven to 350 degrees.

In a large mixing bowl, combine ground chicken, egg, flaxseed, garlic, oregano, red pepper flakes, salt, pepper, and olive oil.

Form into small balls and place in a glass baking dish.

Add ½ inch water to bottom of baking dish.

Bake for 20 minutes.

Turn the meatballs.

Bake another 15–20 minutes.

Enjoy over brown rice, or with brown rice pasta.

NUTRITION INFORMATION ■ **0 G CARBS** ■ **24.25 G PROTEIN** ■ **14.75 G FAT**

SUPER NOTES

Meatballs are one of my favorite things to make because you can do a lot with them. You can add a couple tablespoons of a homemade marinara and place them over zucchini noodles for a faux spaghetti and meatballs, or you can forget the sauce and eat plain. They go great with rice or packed between two slices of bread for a meatball sandwich. They are loaded with protein and I always feel like I'm eating something substantial when I have them. If I'm meal prepping for the week, I'll make meatballs on Sunday and divide them up into a few meals. Just make sure you are using a lean meat, but not the super-lean variety. You don't want them ending up too dry.

SLOW COOKER TURKEY CHILI

*MAKES 4 SERVINGS

1 TEASPOON OLIVE OIL

1 LB. LEAN GROUND TURKEY BREAST

1 MEDIUM YELLOW ONION, PEELED AND DICED

3 CLOVES GARLIC, PEELED AND MINCED

1 RED BELL PEPPER, SEEDED, STEMMED, AND DICED

1 GREEN BELL PEPPER, DICED

1 TOMATO, DICED

1 HATCH GREEN CHILE PEPPER

28 OZ. CAN CRUSHED TOMATOES

15 OZ. CAN TOMATO SAUCE

2½ TEASPOONS CHILI POWDER

½ TEASPOON CUMIN

1 TEASPOON SALT

1 TEASPOON PEPPER

½ TEASPOON CAYENNE

1 CUP KIDNEY BEANS

Brown lean ground turkey breast in olive oil. Drain.

In slow cooker, combine all ingredients with browned turkey.

Cook on low for 8 hours.

NUTRITION INFORMATION ▪ **34 G CARBS** ▪ **27 G PROTEIN** ▪ **11 G FAT**

SUPER NOTES

Chili can be customized in so many ways. I've seen people add potatoes, rice, and more. This is the recipe I like best, but you can alter the seasoning if you like something spicier or milder. If you don't have ground turkey on hand, you can make this chili with a lean ground chicken. There's nothing better than chili on a winter night, right?

LEMON PEPPER BOWL

*MAKES 4 SERVINGS

5 OZ. FRESH SPINACH, STEAMED (5 OZ. FROZEN SPINACH WORKS, TOO)

5 OZ. CORN KERNELS

10 OZ. BROWN RICE

1 TABLESPOON EXTRA-VIRGIN OLIVE OIL

1 POUND SKINLESS CHICKEN BREAST TENDERS

¼ TEASPOON GARLIC POWDER

½ LEMON

SALT

PEPPER

Steam spinach. Drain.

Cook brown rice.

Heat olive oil on medium heat.

Cut chicken into small pieces (about ½ inch) and add to pan with garlic powder, the juice of ½ lemon (I like lots of lemon, so I add a bit more), salt, and lots of pepper.

Cook chicken about 10 minutes or until no longer pink.

In a large mixing bowl, combine chicken, rice, corn, and spinach.

Season with extra salt and pepper to taste.

Enjoy!

NUTRITION INFORMATION ▪ 21 G CARBS ▪ 25 G PROTEIN ▪ 7 G FAT

SUPER NOTES

Rice bowls are a great go-to when you aren't sure what to make. Simply start with some rice (always brown) for your base, and build from there. I love to add grilled peppers and broccoli with grilled chicken, or some bok choy and carrots with wild rice. The possibilities are endless, just pair your favorite veggies with some extra protein and mix it all together. I also recommend keeping frozen vegetables on hand. Fresh always taste better, but sometimes you need something quick and microwavable that is going to fit into your Super Carb equation.

FETA OLIVE WRAP

*MAKES 1 SERVING

4 OZ. GRILLED CHICKEN BREAST

15 G (3–5) KALAMATA OLIVES

1 OZ. FAT-FREE CRUMBLED FETA CHEESE

1 TEASPOON TAHINI

1 ROMAINE LETTUCE LEAF

1 LOW-CARB TORTILLA

Cut chicken and olives into small pieces. Combine ingredients in wrap and enjoy!

NUTRITION INFORMATION ▪ 17 G CARBS ▪ 34 G PROTEIN ▪ 15 G FAT

SUPER NOTES

If you find a low-carb wrap you like, you can get creative for lunches. You're probably used to reaching for the mayo and cheddar when you're making a wrap. Instead, I encourage you to use tahini or hummus as your sauce. They make a great substitute. The Kalamata olives will provide you with a good fat source, and you can always add a little avocado if you want to fatten it up a little more.

CAULIFLOWER "FRIED" RICE

*MAKES 4 SERVINGS

16 OZ. CAULIFLOWER

1 RED BELL PEPPER, SEEDED, STEMMED, AND DICED

1 LARGE CARROT, PEELED AND DICED

½ SWEET ONION, PEELED AND DICED

1 TABLESPOON COCONUT OIL

1 CUP EGG WHITES

LOW SODIUM SOY SAUCE OR BRAGG'S LIQUID AMINOS

1 TEASPOON PEPPER

If you are buying cauliflower whole, separate into small pieces and dice in food processor. Dice about 16 ounces (1 pound) for the recipe.

Heat coconut oil in a large pan on medium heat.

Once hot, add egg whites first, then vegetables.

Stir and cook about 5 minutes.

Add soy sauce and pepper. Stir.

Cook until vegetables are tender.

NUTRITION INFORMATION ■ 13 G CARBS ■ 10 G PROTEIN ■ 4 G FAT

SUPER NOTES

Cauliflower rice has become very popular lately and stores have started expanding with other riced vegetables like broccoli. It's become incredibly convenient for making this dish since you no longer need to pull out the food processor if you buy it already riced. You can also add whatever vegetables you have around the house. I tend to make this toward the end of the week if I have a lot of different veggies that are nearing their expiration. You can mix them all together and make a delicious dish! You can even chop up some skinless chicken breast and mix it in with your rice if you want something more than a side dish. You'll notice I left salt off the ingredient list. That's because soy sauce tends to be so high in sodium that you don't need to add any to it.

EGG WHITE PROTEIN SMOOTHIE

*MAKES 1 SERVING

½ BANANA

1 CUP ALMOND MILK

1 SCOOP EGG WHITE PROTEIN POWDER

1 CUP BABY SPINACH

2 TABLESPOONS PUMPKIN SEEDS

½ CUP ICE

Blend all ingredients together and enjoy!

NUTRITION INFORMATION ▪ **31 G CARBS** ▪ **34 G PROTEIN** ▪ **13 G FAT**

SUPER NOTES

This is a green smoothie recipe that has a good amount of carbs, protein, and fat. It is filling and perfect for when you need a meal-on-the-go. Sometimes there's just not a lot of time to do the cooking you want to do, so a drink like this is all I'll have time for. You can substitute hemp seeds for pumpkin seeds, or mango for banana, but as always, be sure to stay within your numbers if you are substituting. The beauty of a juice or smoothie is that you can mix whatever vegetables, fruits, or seeds you have around the house. The egg white protein powder gives me a nice, lean protein, and I can even mix my vitamins in if I'm making this in the morning.

BISON TACOS

1 TABLESPOON COCONUT OIL

½ MEDIUM ONION, PEELED AND CHOPPED

1 LB. LEAN GROUND BISON

2 TABLESPOONS CHILI POWDER

2 TEASPOONS CUMIN

1 TEASPOON GARLIC POWDER

SALT

PEPPER

1 HEAD ICEBERG LETTUCE

¼ AVOCADO

1 CUP SALSA

Heat coconut oil in skillet on medium heat.

Add onion and bison meat.

Season with chili powder, cumin, garlic powder, salt, and pepper.

Cook until meat is browned.

Wash lettuce and use as shells.

Scoop meat and onion into lettuce.

Top with avocado and salsa.

Enjoy!

NUTRITION INFORMATION ■ 6 G CARBS ■ 25 G PROTEIN ■ 15 G FAT

SUPER NOTES

Tacos are another one of those fantastic and versatile staples for dinner. I always recommend seasoning them yourself. Those taco seasoning mixes at the grocery store are often loaded with salt and sugar. It's not worth it, especially when it's so easy to season on your own. I always have cumin, chili powder, and garlic powder on hand. Fresh herbs are wonderful if you have access. Finally, ground bison is a great alternative to ground beef. It's lower in calories and fat than beef, and it's not as dry as most ground chicken or ground turkey. It does tend to be a bit more expensive than other ground meats, but it's good to know it's out there! Remember, try new foods. You may surprise yourself.

PROTEIN PANCAKES

*MAKES 3 SERVINGS

2 SCOOPS PROTEIN POWDER, VANILLA OR CHOCOLATE

¼ CUP ALMOND FLOUR

½ TEASPOON BAKING POWDER

½ CUP ALMOND MILK

1 TABLESPOON COCONUT OIL

1 TABLESPOON PEANUT BUTTER

Mix protein powder, flour, baking powder, milk, and ½ tablespoon coconut oil.

Heat the other ½ tablespoon of coconut oil over medium heat.

Once hot, add a spoonful of mix.

Cook 1 minute on each side or until brown on edges.

Finish with dollop of peanut butter.

Enjoy!

NUTRITION INFORMATION ▪ 6 G CARBS ▪ 21 G PROTEIN ▪ 13 G FAT

SUPER NOTES

Protein pancakes are a great treat that actually taste like a treat. I make these on the weekend when I have some extra time on my hands since it takes some cleanup (no matter how careful I am, the batter will get everywhere!). Protein powder is a fantastic source of all those amino acids, and there are lots of different things you can do with it. You don't have to JUST mix it with water or milk. You can make pancakes and enjoy a little something special! Plus, you can top with your favorite fruits if you aren't a peanut butter lover. Just remember that fruit is a carb, so keep track of those numbers when you are substituting.

CHICKEN BURRITO

*MAKES 1 SERVING

OLIVE OIL SPRAY

½ YELLOW ONION, PEELED AND CHOPPED

3 OZ. COOKED CHICKEN BREAST, SHREDDED

¼ CUP LOW-SODIUM CANNED BLACK BEANS, DRAINED
AND RINSED

½ SMALL TOMATO, DICED

¼ TEASPOON GROUND CUMIN

¼ TEASPOON CINNAMON

½ TEASPOON CAYENNE

¼ TEASPOON DRY OREGANO

1-10-INCH WHOLE-WHEAT TORTILLA

Spray skillet with olive oil and heat on medium.

Sauté onion for about 5 minutes or until translucent and soft.

Add chicken, beans, tomato, and spices. Mix thoroughly and
heat through.

Spoon mixture into tortilla and wrap.

NUTRITION INFORMATION ▪ 38 G CARBS ▪ 30 G PROTEIN ▪ 8 G FAT

SUPER NOTES

I have a version of this recipe in my book *The Skinny Rules*, where I add ½
cup of unpeeled sweet potato to the recipe. It gives the burrito a nice sweet-
ness and makes it a bit heavier. It's a delicious alternative, but also high in
carbs. To save us some carbs, I removed the sweet potato, and upped the
spices a little to give some added flavor to the chicken.

BOB'S SIGNATURE STIR-FRY

*MAKES 4 SERVINGS

OLIVE OIL SPRAY

6–10 SHIITAKE MUSHROOMS

1 POUND TOTAL OF:

BROCCOLI, CARROTS, ASPARAGUS, SNOW PEAS, JICAMA, AND BEAN SPROUTS

1 TEASPOON RED PEPPER FLAKES

3 GARLIC CLOVES, PEELED AND MINCED

1 TABLESPOON FRESHLY SQUEEZED LIME JUICE

1 POUND SKINLESS CHICKEN BREAST, COOKED

2 CUPS COOKED BROWN RICE

¼ CUP RAW CASHEWS

1 JALAPEÑO, DICED

Spray large skillet with olive oil and heat over medium-high heat.

Sauté mushrooms for 4 minutes.

Toss in the rest of your vegetables along with the red pepper flakes. Cook approximately 5 minutes, stirring occasionally.

Once veggies are tender, toss with lime juice and add cooked chicken breast.

Top the cooked brown rice with mixture, add the cashews and jalapeños before plating, and enjoy!

NUTRITION INFORMATION ▪ 39 G CARBS ▪ 29 G PROTEIN ▪ 8 G FAT

SUPER NOTES

You can substitute the cooked brown rice for wild white rice, or quinoa, depending on what you have on hand. I also like to play around with the protein when I want to change things up. If I'm in the mood for seafood, I'll replace the chicken with shrimp.

TOASTED BREAKFAST

2 SLICES 100% WHOLE-GRAIN BREAD

5.3 OZ. NONFAT PLAIN GREEK YOGURT

1 TABLESPOON OF ALL-NATURAL PEANUT BUTTER

Toast bread.

Spoon yogurt and peanut butter on top of toasted bread and enjoy!

NUTRITION INFORMATION ▪ 40 G CARB ▪ 25 G PROTEIN ▪ 9 G FAT

SUPER NOTES

This is one of my favorite breakfasts! You know I love my nonfat Greek yogurt. The peanut butter is great, but you can also use almond butter, or one of the other nut butters you have around the house. A lot of nut butters are sold as salted or unsalted. This is one of the few meals I can safely get away with using the unsalted without missing much. The Greek yogurt and bread both have sodium in them, so I don't feel like I'm missing much with the unsalted nut butter.

RICE AND KALE MOROCCAN SALAD

1 CUP BARLEY, COOKED

5 CUPS KALE, STEMMED AND CHOPPED

1 RED BELL PEPPER, SEEDED, STEMMED, AND CHOPPED

3 TABLESPOONS LEMON JUICE

2 TABLESPOONS APPLE CIDER VINEGAR

4 CLOVES GARLIC

1 TEASPOON TURMERIC

½ TEASPOON PAPRIKA

3 TABLESPOONS OLIVE OIL

1 TABLESPOON WATER

½ CUP RAW PINE NUTS

SALT

PEPPER

Mix the barley, kale, and bell pepper in a large bowl.

In a food processor, mix lemon juice, vinegar, garlic, turmeric, paprika, olive oil, and water until it becomes a liquid.

Pour liquid over barley, kale, and bell pepper mixture.

Fold in pine nuts and mix.

Add salt and pepper to taste.

NUTRITION INFORMATION ▪ 19 G CARBS ▪ 5 G PROTEIN ▪ 15 G FAT

SUPER NOTES

I spent a lot of years being vegan, so I got used to cooking within that lifestyle. It is difficult to be vegan within the confines of the Super Carb Diet, but it is possible. This Moroccan salad is full of flavor, and you can easily spice it up with some other proteins (chicken breast would be great mixed in instead of the pine nuts). Speaking of spicing it up, your spice cabinet should be one of your best friends during your ninety days on the Super Carb Diet. Don't be afraid to try new seasonings, particularly in salads.

GROUND CHICKEN BOLOGNESE

1 TABLESPOON EXTRA-VIRGIN OLIVE OIL

2 TEASPOONS MINCED GARLIC

3 OZ. CARROT, PEELED AND DICED

1 CELERY STALK, DICED

½ YELLOW ONION, DICED

1 LB. LEAN GROUND CHICKEN

2 TEASPOONS BASIL

1 TEASPOON OREGANO

½ TOMATO, DICED

SALT

PEPPER

Heat olive oil on medium heat.

Sauté garlic, carrot, celery, and onion until tender.

Add ground chicken, seasoning, and tomato.

Cook until meat is brown.

Season with salt and pepper to taste.

Serve over whole-wheat pasta, quinoa pasta, zucchini noodles, or brown rice.

NUTRITION INFORMATION ▪ **4 G CARBS** ▪ **23 G PROTEIN** ▪ **13 G FAT**

SUPER NOTES

This recipe is for the sauce ONLY. You probably know what I'm going to say, but I'll say it anyway: be sure to count the carbs, protein, and fat for whatever noodles you use toward your meal totals. In terms of the cooking, carrots tend to take a while to get tender. If you like them softer, just be sure to cook them longer before putting the chicken in your pan. For your noodles, don't be afraid to experiment with some new options you haven't tried before. Zucchini noodles are great if you want to avoid large amounts of carbs, but they don't have quite the same taste as the other noodles. Brown rice pasta is one of my favorites, but I know that I need to eat it right away. When you refrigerate brown rice pasta, it loses a lot of its moisture over time, so it doesn't reheat as well as traditional pasta. Whole-wheat pasta is the most like white pasta in terms of taste, in my opinion, but it's the most carb-heavy of all the options. If you choose that, you may be reaching your carb limits quicker than you want to.

ITALIAN WEDDING SOUP

*MAKES 8 SERVINGS

MEATBALLS:

- 1.5 LB. LEAN GROUND TURKEY
- 2 CLOVES GARLIC, PEELED AND MINCED
- 2 EGG WHITES
- ¼ CUP GRATED PARMESAN CHEESE
- SALT
- PEPPER

SOUP:

- 1 TEASPOON OLIVE OIL
- 1 CUP CARROTS, DICED
- 1 CUP CELERY, DICED
- 1 CLOVE GARLIC, MINCED
- 1 YELLOW ONION, CHOPPED
- 1 QUART LOW SODIUM CHICKEN BROTH
- 1 QUART UNSALTED CHICKEN STOCK
- 1 TEASPOON OREGANO
- 12 OZ. FROZEN SPINACH

Combine all meatball ingredients and roll into balls. Set aside.

In a large pot, heat olive oil and sauté carrots, celery, garlic, and onion over medium heat.

When carrots soften, add broth, stock, and seasonings.

Once liquid is boiling, add meatballs and spinach.

Cook until meatballs are done.

NUTRITION INFORMATION ▪ **4 G CARBS** ▪ **22.4 G PROTEIN** ▪ **3 G FAT**

SUPER NOTES

This version omits the noodles that are in a lot of other versions. You can add some if they fit within your numbers, but I don't think you will miss them with the meatballs and veggies. You'll notice I just said to add the broth when the carrots soften. Carrots take forever to soften. Or maybe I'm just impatient. Either way, they will still cook once you add the broth, but to get the right texture, don't add until you notice them softening a bit.

P.S. You can also do this in a crock pot. You'll have to mix the meatballs ahead of time, but then you can add everything to the pot and leave it cooking for the day. Your house will smell delicious!

ROTISSERIE CHICKEN

*SERVING SIZE: 3 OUNCES

1 WHOLE CHICKEN (ABOUT 3 POUNDS)

1 TABLESPOON PAPRIKA

¼ CUP OLIVE OIL

¼ CUP CHICKEN STOCK

3 CLOVES GARLIC, MINCED

SALT

PEPPER

Remove the neck/giblets from the chicken and pat dry.

Salt the inside of the chicken.

Mix paprika, olive oil, chicken stock, garlic, and desired amount of salt and pepper.

Place chicken on the rotisserie and cook on high for 10–12 minutes.

Use the paprika mix to baste chicken.

Alter heat to medium temperature and close lid of grill.

Cook 1–1½ hours or until the internal temperature of the chicken reaches 180 degrees, basting about every 20 minutes.

Let cool and enjoy!

NUTRITION INFORMATION ■ 0 G CARBS ■ 15 G PROTEIN ■ 12 G FAT

SUPER NOTES

Rotisserie chicken is SO EASY. You need to have the right equipment, but if you do, you're all set to make one. I like a rotisserie chicken because you can take the skin off and use the meat throughout the week for soups, salads, or any dish that needs a lean protein. This recipe includes a basting mix that will give your bird some nice flavor, but if you want to have a more plain-tasting chicken, simply baste with oil and omit the stock, garlic, and paprika. That way you can season the meat later when you add it to your other dishes. If you don't have a roaster, you can purchase great whole ro-tisserie chickens at most grocery stores, fully cooked. I noticed there's lots of rotisserie chickens that are flavored at the grocery (BBQ, lemon pepper, etc.). If you are buying one cooked, read the labels to ensure you aren't get-ting one that has been roasted with tons of sugar or other additives.

FINAL THOUGHTS

You've taken the steps to make positive changes in your life. I'm proud of each and every one of you, and I'll be excited to hear from all of you after you complete the Super Carb Diet. Remember to let me know how you're doing. Show me your progress. Tweet me (@MyTrainerBob). I also want to see those before-and-after selfies on Instagram, so be sure to use #SuperCarb Diet when you're uploading those beautiful pics.

When I had my heart attack in February of 2017, I wasn't sure what was next. I faced depression and anxiety like I never had before. What followed was a journey that made me stronger and healthier than ever. My professional focus has always been to get other people to lose weight. I still want to do that, but now it's not just about the weight. I need you all to be strong enough to survive anything that comes your way, because I know life is going to throw some tough shit at you.

They say everything happens for a reason. My heart attack provided me an opportunity to start from scratch. I'm much more appreciative of my health and happiness. I was given new resources that opened my eyes to philosophies I had never considered. The Super Carb Diet is everything I learned from that experience, as well as all my previous years in the health-and-fitness industry. Crafting this diet gave me a new purpose. I'm so excited to share it with all of you so you can be healthier than ever, and strong enough to fight off whatever comes your way. Life is a gift. Put the work in now so you can enjoy unwrapping it.

ACKNOWLEDGMENTS

First and foremost, I want to thank Danny Pellegrino, my ghostwriter. I have had the best experience working with you. You're an incredibly talented person and such a good friend. You make me laugh all the time. I love you.

Thanks to Elizabeth Beier at St. Martin's. I sat in your office when I was shopping this book because I wanted to change things up, and I am so thrilled that I did. You get me and you understand me. Also, thanks to the rest of the top-notch team at St. Martin's. I am so happy to work with such a wonderful group of forward thinkers.

Thank you to Richard Abate, my book agent. I love the way your brain works.

Nicole Trinler, you are my right- and left-hand "person," who has worked tirelessly on this book, keeping me on schedule (which is NOT an easy thing to do).

On a personal note, I would also like to thank a very special group of people who were present during the time of my heart attack, and without whom I would not be here. Thank you to Dr. Hazem Shoirah, a doctor who wasn't even supposed to be at the gym the day of my attack, but who was there and went into action immediately. Dr. Z saved my life.

Thanks to Sean Stevens, my friend. You were there with me that day and immediately went into action mode.

And to Sherry Ward, the coach at the gym who got the AED off the wall and brought it to me.

The paramedics with Engine 3 in New York that got my heart beating and got me to the hospital so quickly.

Thank you to Dr. Gowda at Beth Israel Hospital and the FANTASTIC staff there that took such good care of me.

To the unbelievable Cardiac Rehab team at The Rusk Institute in New York, you all not only helped with my heart, you helped with my mind, too.

Of course, I have to thank my dog, Karl, who walked with me every day in the city when I didn't want to walk with anyone else. It was just the two of us out there on the streets. I love him SO much.

Finally, I want to thank Whitney Houston and everyone involved in making *The Bodyguard*. One night in the hospital, I was so shell-shocked and depressed about what had happened to me, Anthony got the nurses to bring in a DVD player, and we watched *The Bodyguard* while eating peanut butter and jelly sandwiches (the only thing I would eat). It was the best night ever. No matter how bad life gets, just put on that movie and it will make everything right with the world.

To everyone I mentioned (and all of you reading at home), *I hope life treats you kind. And I hope you have all you've dreamed of. And I wish you joy and happiness . . .*

But above all this, I wish you love.

NOTES

Introduction: "Body by Bob"

1. The Miriam-Webster Definition of carbohydrate. https://www.merriam
   -webster.com/dictionary/carbohydrate
2. Xu JQ, Murphy SL, Kochanek KD, Bastian, BA. "Deaths: Final data for
   2013," *National Vital Statistics Report* (2016):64(2). https://www.cdc.gov
   /nchs/data/nvsr/nvsr64/nvsr64_02.pdf

1: "Carbs Don't Make You Fat"

1. Karl, J. Philip et al. "Substituting whole grains for refined grains in a
   6-wk randomized trial favorably affects energy-balance metrics in healthy
   men and postmenopausal women," *The American Journal of Clinical Nutrition*, February 8, 2017. http://ajcn.nutrition.org/content/early/2017/02/07
   /ajcn.116.139683
2. Caponnolo, A. et al. "Non-Celiac Gluten Sensitivity among Patients Per-
   ceiving Gluten-Related Symptoms." Accessed at PubMed.gov, https://www
   .ncbi.nlm.nih.gov/pubmed/26043918
3. Fairfield, Hannah. "Factory Food," *The New York Times*, April 3, 2010.
   http://nytimes.com/2010/04/04/business/04metrics.html

2: "The Plan"

1. Block, Jason P. et al. "Consumers' estimation of calorie content at fast food restaurants: cross sectional observational study," May 23, 2013. http://www.bmj.com/content/346/bmj.f2907.

2. National Heart, Lung, and Blood Institute, "How Much Sleep Is Enough?" https://www.nhlbi.nih.gov/health/health-topics/topics/sdd/howmuch

3: "Good Carbs"

1. Goodman, Jack. "Grocery Shopping: Who, Where and When," The Time Use Institute, October 2008. http://timeuseinstitute.org/Grocery%20White%20Paper%202008.pdf

2. Jonnalagadda, Satya S. et al. "Putting the Whole Grain Puzzle Together: Health Benefits Associated with Whole Grains—Summary of American Society for Nutrition 2010 Satellite Symposium," *The Journal of Nutrition*. http://wholegrainscouncil.org/sites/default/files/atoms/files/ASNsummary2010.pdf

4: "Carbage"

1. Diabetes. http://www.who.int/mediacentre/factsheets/fs312/en/

5: "All About Protein"

1. "Eggs," National Heart Foundation of Australia. https://www.heartfoundation.org.au/healthy-eating/food-and-nutrition/protein-foods/eggs

2. Siepmann, T. et al. "Hypogonadism and erectile dysfunction associated with soy product consumption." https://www.ncbi.nlm.nih.gov/pubmed/21353476

3. http://www.consumerreports.org/cro/magazine-archive/2010/july/food/protein-drinks/what-our-tests-found/index.htm

7: "Lettuce Talk More About Vegetables"

1. "Vegetable Subgroups." https://www.isbe.net/Documents/vegetable-subgroups.pdf Also see: "Dietary Guidelines for Americans 2010," U.S. Department of Agriculture. https://health.gov/dietaryguidelines/dga2010/DietaryGuidelines2010.pdf

2. McLaughlin, August. "What Are the Benefits of Starchy Vegetables?" *SFGate*. http://healthyeating.sfgate.com/benefits-starchy-vegetables-2259.html

10: "Sleeping Your Way to Healthy"

1. "A Twin Study of Sleep Duration and Body Mass Index." https://www.ncbi.nlm.nih.gov/pmc/articles/PMC2823270/

2. St.-Onge, Marie-Pierre et al. Short sleep duration increases energy intakes but does not change energy expenditure in normal-weight individuals. http://ajcn.nutrition.org/content/early/2011/06/29/ajcn.111.013904

13: "Aging"

1. Janssen I, R. Ross. "Linking age-related changes in skeletal muscle mass and composition with metabolism and disease." *The Journal of Nutrition, Health & Aging*, Nov.–Dec. 2005; 9(6):408–419. http://www.ncbi.nlm.uih.gov/entrez/query
2. "Childhood Obesity Facts," Centers for Disease Control and Prevention. https://www.cdc.gov/healthyschools/obesity/facts.htm Also see: Cheryl D. Fryar et al., *Prevalence of Overweight and Obesity Among Children and Adolescents Aged 2–19 Years: United States, 1963–1965 Through 2013–2014* (Atlanta, GA: National Center for Health Statistics, 2014).
3. The North American Menopause Society. https://www.menopause.org/for-women/menopauseflashes/menopause-symptoms-and-treatments

17: "Frequently Asked Questions"

1. "Heart Attack Symptoms in Women," American Heart Association. http://www.heart.org/HEARTORG/Conditions/HeartAttack/WarningSignsofaHeartAttack/Heart-Attack-Symptoms-in-Women_UCM_436448_Article.jsp#.WQjmH1Pysk8

"Fitness"

1. Reynolds, Gretchen. "Carbs During Workouts May Fend Off Colds," *The New York Times*, December 7, 2016. https://mobile.nytimes.com/2016/12/07/well/move/carbs-during-workouts-may-fend-off-colds.html
2. "Learn About Automated External Defibrillators," American Red Cross. http://www.redcross.org/prepare/location/workplace/easy-as-aed
3. "35 CPR Statistics," *Journal of Emergency Medical Services*. http://www.jems.com/galleries/2013/07/35-cpr-statistics.html

INDEX